I dedicate this book to my darling Richard for being the first man who has ever loved me as a woman should be loved and for giving me the confidence to love myself. You have changed my life and I just can't thank you enough.

This book is also dedicated to everyone whose lives have been affected by brain tumours.

Acknowledgements

Firstly, I would like to thank the man who helped me make this book come together and for believing that I had a story to tell. It's been a hard eight months and this guy never gave up on me – even though he probably wished he had as I hardly gave him a minute's peace! I think he will be going into rehab now. So, thank you, Douglas, I owe all this to you. This is my dream come true. You have found a friend for life.

I also want to thank my mum, Margaret, and dad, Rob, who were always there for me, never gave up on me and, however hard things got, never stopped loving me. It is because of you both that I am still here today.

Thanks also to Michael, Robina, Dorothy and Averil for putting up with your mad sister all these years. The rest of my family – thank you all so much. There are just too many to name you all.

I also want to thank the people who helped me get here today – my surgeons: Mr Currie, Mr Blaiklock and Mr Fouyas. These men are the most highly skilled I know and, yes, they did all say there was a brain in my head. Thanks, also, to all the other doctors and nurses at ward 40, in Foresterhill Hospital, Aberdeen, who have helped me. I am sorry for being the world's worst patient. Dr Tom Heneghan – who was my GP from the start – any time, night or day, you were always there for me and explained things to me in a way I could understand.

To the Scottish News of the World, thank you also. You are all ace.

Also to my best friend, Anwen, though we have only known each other for three years, you made me see what a true friend really is.

I want to thank the girls who did my hair and make up for the book's front cover. I can't take the credit for it, so thank you to Donna Murray and Sarah Main, at Hair Design 101 in Lossiemouth and to Mark Williamson for doing my photos.

Last one I promise! To Marie Stevenson at Lipstick Publishing, thank you for everything.

Foreword
By Richard Blood

It's not everyday a stranger comes up to me in the street and blatantly chats me up, believe me. Therefore, when Caroline first confronted me, I was surprised and intrigued in equal measure. She hit me with a line that we'd met the previous night. Her directness caught me off guard and interested me enough to want to see her again.

Just twenty-four hours later, I was to see another side of Caroline's unique personality. Arriving at her mother's house to take her out on our date, I was not prepared when she greeted me with a quick one-two of put-downs – criticising my ironing skills and commenting how old I looked out of uniform. On any other night, I might have turned on my heel but I grudgingly had to admit that, at least, she was being consistent. Her bluntness had impressed me one minute, and then mildly insulted me the next!

Maybe it's the masochist in me, but I was intrigued to see what would happen. Until that day, I'd never met a girl who could surprise and infuriate simultaneously. That was three years ago and, to be honest, I'm still sticking around to see what will happen next.

One thing you can guarantee with Caroline is she never fails to leave a first impression. Rarely pausing to worry about what people think, she steams in and says whatever is on her mind. With such forwardness, she can talk her way into any job and never struggles to make friends.

The flipside, however, is that sometimes her bluntness can rub others up the wrong way. People, not used to someone so outspoken, often can't handle her directness and it counts against her. Yet, the great thing about Caroline is she never lets anything get to her. I guess when you've lived your life with a life-threatening condition hanging over you, the little things that upset most people hardly register.

One of the things that most impressed me about Caroline was her attitude to her condition. I imagined someone living with such a condition would have a permanent link to emergency help. Caroline, however, takes it all in her stride. She treats her tumour in the same way she would any other minor irritation, like the rest of us treat a stone in our shoe. The only difference is, sadly, she cannot remove the foreign body in her head quite so easily.

When Caroline was only ten, her doctors feared she may never grow up. Physically smaller than other children, they worried her brain tumour might affect her growth hormones. However, although she eventually put on the inches, in some ways, Caroline is still that little girl. Fussed over for most of her life, with doctors at her beck and call, it's natural she expects a certain level of attention.

I think most of us might have preconceived ideas about how someone who has suffered a life of near constant health problems should be. We might expect them to be fragile and delicate, someone we should tiptoe around.

Caroline, on the other hand, is strong-willed, outspoken and someone who gets straight to the point. Ever since she was a young girl, she's had to fight for her life and shout to be heard. For her, life is too short not to say what's on her mind. Behind that tough exterior, however, she is a caring soul and always thinks of others before herself. Opening up their life for all to see is not everyone's choice but Caroline hopes that, by laying bare her experiences, someone else might draw comfort. That's the type of person she is. All I ask is that, before you judge her, just put yourself in her position for one day and ask "How would I deal with this?"

CONTENTS

Introduction

The tension was unbearable. Standing on the start line, I glanced nervously from side to side. Around me, the other children were pacing up and down on the spot, shaking their legs to get the circulation going on this fresh spring morning. Going by the seriousness of their expressions, you would have thought they were limbering up for the Olympic 100m sprint final, instead of the Primary One 40m dash at Mortlach School Annual Sports Day, in the Scottish highlands.

Ahead of me, the chalk-lined lanes seemed to stretch off into the distance as I looked once more along the rows of excited faces on the trackside. I picked out mum one last time, standing up near the finish, where I'd imagined myself breaking the line a hundred times over in my head. Smiling broadly, she gave me the thumbs up. Then the Sports teacher called for silence.

"On your marks, get set, go."

With that, we were off, wind rushing in our faces, the yells of our parents ringing in our ears. I could feel the adrenalin flowing through my body as I willed it to push on to the finishing tape.

Out of the corners of my eyes, I could see my competitors edging in front on both sides. Soon, I didn't need to squint. They were clearly leaving me behind, bouncing away like gazelles. In contrast, I was hobbling along, my gait so awkward it would have been a sin to call it running. My right leg was turned in to my left, my back arched and my head was angled to the sky. I tried to summon an energy boost to get me back in the race but it was clear there would be no surge of speed. I was trailing. Panicked, I looked around. All the children were in front of me. I was last. I looked up to the crowd at the side – everyone transfixed on the action ahead. Only one pair of eyes was on me. Mum was still smiling and waving her arms furiously, willing me to catch the others. In her eyes though, I could see her panic.

Starting school early at the age of four, I was always going to be physically weaker than my classmates were, so perhaps it was ambitious to think I had a chance of winning my first school sprint. However, this was no defeat; it was a mauling. I trailed home in what seemed like an eternity after the others and it was only then the other parents spotted me. They shot pitying glances between mum and me, continuing to heap praise or commiserations on their own kids.

Mum didn't say a word. She didn't have to. The effects of what she'd witnessed went far deeper than the casual disappointment that her child had been beaten in a race. She knew something serious was wrong with me. That moment, when I stood on the start line, was the last time mum would be able to look upon me as she would any other little girl.

The following years would see my health deteriorate, almost to the point of death, before surgeons discovered a tumour growing in my brain. I owe my life to their expertise but have had to live with the fear that the ticking time bomb in my head could claim my life at any point.

On the day I was finally diagnosed, I ceased being solely Caroline, a girl with her life ahead of her. I didn't know it then, but it was the day I became "That Tumour Girl", a child dependent on medical attention for the rest of her life. I lived in fear, terrified of going to sleep in case I did not wake up. My behaviour baffled doctors and pushed my family to the brink of insanity.

While other children's memories are of first days at school, birthday parties and fairy tale Christmases, mine are of starched hospital bed sheets, the pungent smell of clinical disinfectant and having my hair clipped to assist surgery.

There was nothing I wanted more than for surgeons to cut the foreign body out of my skull, give me my life back and take me back to the little girl standing on the start line on that spring morning in Dufftown, the place where I grew up. The tumour dominated my entire being and, in my mind, I exaggerated its influence; not only the physical presence it occupied in my head but also the heavy burden it placed on my emotional state. I used to think of it as a death sentence and spent my days, and most of my nights, in sheer panic wondering when my life would end.

Despite the trauma, however, I am one of the lucky ones. It has been sixteen years since I learned I was living with a tumour and I am still here to tell my story. Others, as you will learn in this book, have not been so fortunate. Brain tumours, whether aggressively cancerous or less so, have a devastating effect on sufferers and the loved ones whose lives they touch. The statistics tell their own story. Brain cancer kills more children and young adults than leukaemia and meningitis combined and, if current trends continue, it could become the number one killer of children in the next decade.

My surgeons diagnosed me with an inoperable, low-grade astrocytoma and, on the cancer scale of one to four, it was on the lower end. That fact saved my life and allowed me to live as I have. For many children diagnosed with an inoperable malignant brain tumour, they will only stand a 25% chance of surviving five years.

Samantha Dickson, whose parents Neil and Angela set up a charity to aid research into brain cancers, died just days after her sixteenth birthday, on 31st October 1996, after a brave two-year battle.

When doctors told my parents the dreadful news about my condition, they advised them to take me home and prepare for the worst. Yet, here I am. I am not the only person who knows what it's like to live with a brain tumour and I won't be the last. However, I want people to know what it's like dealing with such a serious condition day in, day out. I hope my story offers some hope to those recently introduced to the complexities of this condition and, for those who have never given brain tumours a second thought, maybe it will give an insight into what can still be a taboo subject.

If one person living with a serious medical affliction takes a crumb of comfort from my experience – even if it's to thank their lucky stars they didn't grow up in a household with me in it – then it will all have been worthwhile.

So put your feet up and switch off Eastenders and Coronation Street because – after you have read my story – you will see my life is a soap opera to rival the best.

Chapter One
Go Home and Take a Paracetamol

As soon as I woke I knew instinctively I was in trouble. It took an age to open my eyelids and the light, although dimmed through the curtains, pierced through my retinas like a laser beam. My head throbbed with a dull, pulsing pain. This was not that unusual. From the age of five, I had been used to living with almost constant headaches. At this point, aged nineteen, for me to notice these immediately started the alarm bells ringing.

I reached a hand to my head, pinching the temples of my skull. I then slowly stroked my hair round to the back of my neck, as if my fingers would be able to detect the root of the problem. I began probing the base of my skull. I could feel the shunt – a valve and pipe fitted into the back of my head when I was five that links to my stomach to relieve my hydrocephalus, or water on the brain. It seemed normal, but then how could I tell whether the artificial drainage system was working inside my head simply by pressing a few digits here and there?

No, something was definitely up. I tried to look around my bedroom but the furniture was blurry. This was no common or garden early morning head fog. This had to be more serious. I tried to lift my eyes in the direction of the window but the closer I got to the room's source of light, the more painful it was for me to look.

What was going on? The shunt was not my only concern. For eleven years I'd known a tumour had been growing on my brain. After it was discovered, the surgeons had told me it was inoperable and removing it could leave me paralysed. That was the good news. What they also said was that leaving it could one day kill me. Was that day today?

Slowly I began to get my bearings. I was at my eldest sister Robina's house in New Elgin, Morayshire, where I'd been living for a few months. Robina had moved up from Dufftown with her six-year-old son, Kyle, and was a nurse in the local hospital. Today she had left early for a weekend visiting friends in Glasgow. It was Saturday and she was going to be away all weekend. I was alone in the three-bedroom house.

I tried to remember what had happened. I had been out with a few friends the night before in nearby Elgin. I avoid alcohol mainly because of my condition, so the two Cokes I drank would hardly have been responsible for these headaches. I managed to get up but the throbbing in my skull was relentless. Getting dressed was an arduous task. Even lifting my head up straight seemed an effort. Trying to squeeze my head through the hole in a sweater was agony so I thought better of it and switched to a cardigan. I nibbled on a bit of toast and slumped on the sofa.

The shunt had blocked twice before but, since the pipe had been lengthened three years earlier, things had been fine.

I must have blacked out because when I next came round on the sofa, it was an hour later. The throbbing pain was still constant and, although it was nearly midday on a summer's day in June, I still had the curtains drawn because the prospect of daylight was too much for my eyes. I telephoned my three sisters but, strange as it may seem, they weren't overly concerned. When you've been dealing with someone with a brain tumour for eleven years you become immune to hearing about headaches. Even mum, who always came running to my side but had recently left to start a new life for herself in Spain, wanted a second opinion before jumping on the next plane home.

In desperate need of some sympathy, I called my then boyfriend Stuart. He was in the RAF, was six years older than me and made me feel secure. He stepped up to the plate straight away, came round, got me together and rushed me down to the hospital. The last thing I wanted was to interact with the outside world but he was right – I had to see a doctor. In the waiting room, near Ward Seven where Robina usually worked, there were only three chairs. Luckily there were two free. I eyed up the other patient, each of us checking if the other was truly ill enough to bother our over-stretched medics on a weekend.

Clearly though, the doctor had been having one of those days. Either that or he had a pressing engagement somewhere else and he was just trying to clear the decks before shutting up shop for the day. Whatever the reason, he couldn't have been less concerned than if I had said my hand was sore where my grocery bag had cut into it.

Despite being given a crash course into brain tumours, shunts and the effects of pressure on the head, the doctor dismissed me with the helpful advice to go home, take a paracetamol and rest up. Instinctively, I wanted a second opinion but I was too weary to argue. Stuart took me home, nursed me on the sofa and left me to hopefully sleep it off. In need of comfort, I shunned the single bed Robina had kindly offered me when I'd moved in three months previously, choosing instead her much more comfy double divan.

If I thought Saturday was bad, it was a picnic compared to how I was on Sunday morning. By now my head felt like a lead weight, my eyes would only open half way and it felt like someone was battering the inside of my skull with an iron bar. I rang for the cavalry but Robina, still living it up in the big city, was not convinced my situation merited her cutting short a long weekend. I can't blame her. It's hard to overrule a so-called expert when a doctor has dismissed it as a twenty-four hour thing. Luckily I had Stuart by my side. As I lay on the sofa, I was aware he was talking but I couldn't respond. He later told me I'd had a petit mal, a small epileptic seizure and common by-product of the brain surgery I had endured as a youngster. But, although I was drifting in and out of consciousness, suffering seizures, black-outs and feeling nauseous, hardly any of it seemed out of place to him, or my family, because of my condition and poor health record. I knew, however, that something definitely was not right. I gave it another night to fully exhaust the doc's prescription of paracetamol and rest, but by Monday morning I had not improved.

I managed to get up but by now, I could only wear sunglasses in the house; the exposure to daylight was causing unbearable pain. I knew ringing Stuart again was out of the question because he was on guard duty at the RAF base in Lossiemouth. RAF men were only to be excused for wives and immediate family. I did not fall into that category.

I endeavoured to rest a little in bed before taking myself off to my doctor but the day slipped away from me and, before I knew, I was waking up to evening twilight. The house was still deserted. Summoning all the energy I could muster, I phoned the out-of-hours service again. Confused and dazed, I struggled to explain the medical factors playing a part in my poor state. The nurse must have thought she was dealing with someone who'd enjoyed a liquid lunch and dinner. I pleaded for a doctor to make a house call but she, like the doctor, told me to pop a couple of painkillers and I'd be right as rain. In desperation, I complained I was alone and there was no paracetamol in the house. Showing the compassion for which our health service is renowned, she helpfully suggested I take myself along to my local petrol station – it would surely stock them.

Close to tears, I collapsed on the bed. This was it, I thought. The tumour, which had been growing on the stem of my brain for the last decade, had now taken over my mind and I would lose my faculties one by one. Either that, or the shunt designed to relieve pressure caused by the growth, had blocked causing my head to expand to the point it would pop like a water balloon. I was sure this was how it was going to end: alone in a house, with my family miles away.

I stirred from my slumber at the sound of a voice. It was Robina. I was so relieved to see her and to know I was still alive that I hadn't appreciated it was now Tuesday morning, a full three days since I'd started feeling unwell. Yet my elation must have masked my symptoms because my sister, unimpressed that I was still in my bed, announced she was going to work. As the door slammed behind her, I determined to take matters into my own hands. I reached for the phone to call my doctor but by now the numbers on the telephone had blurred into one and I couldn't even dial 999 for an ambulance.

After dressing, I staggered into the street, shielding my eyes from the light and almost bent double trying to stop the pain behind my eyes. All I could think of was getting to hospital. I stumbled into a Post Office and managed to blurt out what was going on. Luckily, the owner phoned for a taxi that rushed me to the local hospital. Yet, even after checking myself in, it was six hours before doctors agreed to a brain scan to assess what was going on. Stuck in casualty, all I had for nourishment was a packet of cheese and onion crisps while lying on a trolley.

4

Robina appeared again, after I'd managed to collar a nurse to ask her to alert my sister. Now, she was horrified to see my complaints had come to this. She was stunned at the seriousness and scolded herself for not acting sooner.

When the scan finally confirmed my shunt was blocked, the penny dropped and they conceded I was an urgent case and announced I was to be rushed to Aberdeen Royal Infirmary for emergency surgery. The trip from Elgin to Aberdeen, never a good one at the best of times along the tortuously slow A96, was a blur. I recall being admitted into the emergency ward and being hurriedly run through the procedure before the lights went out completely.

When I came to properly, sometime later I was amazed; first, to be able to stare into the glaring hospital ward lights without feeling sick and second, to be greeted by a relieved Robina and my dad, Rob. Surgeons had performed an emergency operation to relieve the blockage and fit a new shunt. If the build-up of fluid had got much worse, I would have died. Mum arrived shortly after; she had caught the first available flight back once she had heard.

"That was close," Robina said.

You're telling me, I thought.

Chapter Two
Meet the Family

Even by today's standards, I have a pretty unusual family. As I never tire of telling everybody and much to the chagrin of my mum, I am in the privileged position of having one mother, three dads, three sisters, and 13 half or step brothers and sisters. My clan doesn't so much have a family tree but a rather unkempt bush. We're not the only family to have experienced the dissolution of marriages and the blossoming of new relationships but where I think we differ from most broods is how well we still manage to get on with each other despite all this.

With our extended relations, you could imagine it would be like World War Three if we all came together but, for the most part, we all seem to tolerate each other's lifestyles. We might not be a great advert for the institution of marriage but, hey, it could be a hell of a lot worse.

Things didn't start out that way, though. My nana and grandpa (Dorothy and Robin Weir) lived a long and happy life together. In 1948, three years after the war, they had followed nana's parents, John and Peggy Urquhart, when they left Paisley in Renfrewshire (on mainland Scotland) to start a new life on the Isle of Skye, the largest of the Inner Hebrides.

John, a retired police officer, had become a café shop owner in Paisley after hanging up his baton but was looking for a fresh challenge and a new way of life in a country still taking stock of itself after five long years of fighting. Knowing the island well after spending many a summer on the west coast, he settled with Peggy in Portree, the island's capital on the north east side. The islanders did not know it, but John was something of a pioneer in his day, bringing with him the first ice cream on Skye, made from a secret recipe he gleaned from an Italian friend back home. Armed with his precious commodity, my great-granddad swiftly opened up the island's first ice cream parlour in Portree harbour.

Known as the "misty isle" because of its traditional murky weather, Skye has been enchanting visitors for centuries. The evocative legend of Bonnie Prince Charlie and Flora Macdonald – the local girl whose heroics safeguarded the young pretender's flight from the mainland after his defeat at Culloden in 1746 – has secured the island's romantic place in the nation's heart. A land of contrasts, its reputation for inclement weather belies the gorgeous summer sunshine that can make you think you're in the Caribbean, and its tawny moorland gives way to rugged slopes of the breathtaking Cuillin Hills.

The lure of the island proved too much for recently wed nana and Robin and they followed some six years later. For Robin, born in Malaysia to an Australian mother who sent him to Glasgow for an education, he relished the opportunity to trade the hustle and bustle of an over-congested central belt for the serenity of the western isles. Joined by Dorothy's brother Ian and his wife, the young couples set to work quickly building a business for the family and giving something back to the isle that had given them their home. Taking over a derelict site in Portree's High Street, they renovated it to establish the Caledonian Hotel, complete with café and chip shop underneath.

Not the type to rest on their laurels, they soon sold the now bustling hotel and set their sights on a bigger opportunity. Situated on an inlet just east of the town's harbour was the Cuillin Hills Hotel, commanding unparalleled views of the famous mountain range. A former hunting lodge once used by Lord Macdonald of the Isles, it had been utilised during the war as a temporary home for people evacuated from the mainland. A local hotelier then took over the building and transformed it into a top class hotel but sadly never lived long enough to run it. That's when my grandparents took it over. Running the nineteen bedroom hotel was a full time job, especially after the extensions the family added on in the 1960s.

By that time nana was also trying to raise three children. Her two sons had been born at home in Paisley before the move north. My mother Margaret was the youngest, born on Christmas Day in 1955, much to the delight of her big brothers. Nana gave birth to Margaret in the house, a newly built cottage just yards from the hotel near the inlet of Scorrybreck. The two boys were told Santa had brought them a little sister but so ecstatic were they, that the ensuing years they expected more of the same. It was a magical time for Margaret and the boys, growing up with their cousins as neighbours and best friends. The family branched out and took advantage of the local Forestry Commission's decision to release land near the hotel. Margaret's brothers soon built houses on the hillside overlooking the bay next to their parents' home.

For mum, life has gone full circle and she is now back working in the hotel trade on Skye. Back then, however, she showed her determination of spirit by rejecting the family business, deciding instead to pursue a career in nursing. Without any formal training, she secured a job at the local hospital aged just seventeen and it was while planning her new career she met a local banker called Archie Nicolson. He was nineteen and, after a relatively short courtship, they married two years later at, appropriately enough, the family hotel. There was no getting away from the place when they moved into a house in the grounds of the old building shortly afterwards, and for a while things seemed to be going well for the young couple embarking down the road of life together.

Mum gave birth to their first daughter Robina a year later and they were soon looking forward to a new challenge when Archie's job with the bank was transferred to Dufftown, in Morayshire.

"If Rome was built on seven hills, then Dufftown was built on seven stills." So goes the local saying about Scotland's self-proclaimed home of whisky. Founded in 1817 by James Duff, 4th Earl of Fife, the highland town was initially named Balvenie. The Earl started the building of Dufftown to provide employment after the Napoleonic Wars but the surrounding hills' perfect water sources made it the ideal location to set up the country's busiest legal and illegal distilleries nearly two centuries ago. Today the town may not boast the seven distilleries but it still produces some of the world's most famous names in Scotch like Glenfiddich, Glenlivet and Balvenie. These days the centre is still dominated by a tower, housing a clock that led to the execution of a little-known Scots 'Robin

Hood' called MacPherson of Kingussie. This infamous free-booter was condemned to death at Banff in 1700 for robbing the rich and giving to the poor. A local petition was raised to spare his life but while the pardon was on its way, MacPhersons' arch-enemy Lord Braco – unfortunately the Sheriff of Banff – put the clock forward an hour to make sure he would hang. Many years later, the clock was removed from Banff and to this day stares down on the good folk of Dufftown.

It was here mum and dad came to live, moving into a semi-detached cottage. Sharing a garden with the family next door meant my parents quickly got to know their neighbours Rob and Elsie Macdonald in Fern Cottage, who had a son Michael, and the foursome quickly became firm friends.

The arrival of second daughter Dorothy in 1979 added to the family but Archie grew disillusioned with the bank and persuaded mum to uproot for the second time in just 18 months. He took her back to Skye and the Cuillin Hills Hotel. Although mum had turned her back on the unpredictable hotel trade, Archie wanted to give it a go and they moved in with nana and grandpa while dad learned the ropes.

Mum and dad still kept in touch with the Macdonalds in Dufftown but their concern for Elsie grew when she developed heart problems and doctors scheduled her for a bypass operation.

At that time, mum was pregnant with yours truly and I duly entered the world on 13th December 1981. Like all mum's babies, I was a breach birth but, as a result of additional complications, I was delivered by caesarean section in hospital at Inverness. Margaret was only told afterwards she'd haemorrhaged in theatre and undergone blood transfusions to get her count back up.

Four months after I was born, Elsie went into hospital in Aberdeen for the bypass operation. She seemed to recover well from the surgery and was looking forward to the day she could go home from hospital. That day never came, however, because she suddenly developed problems and died less than a week later. The following day, mum, received a letter from the hospital written by Elsie just hours before she died saying how much she was looking forward to seeing her again. It broke

9

mum's heart. Elsie was only 39. In the months that followed mum tried to offer as much support to Rob as she could, often travelling the 160 miles to Dufftown with the three of us girls to help him get over his grief.

Obviously, I can't remember too much about my life at that point but by all accounts, I was a near perfect baby who slept for hours. Although, as mum points out, I must have been storing sleep for the torture I would put the family through in later years.

Only one small episode, at the age of one, caused the family slight anxiety. During a routine check-up, our health visitor noticed something not quite right with my eyes; a slight squint, which only presented itself occasionally. Confused, she asked for a second opinion and referred me to Inverness to consult an eye specialist. The results came back negative. Mum was relieved I seemed to have nothing far wrong with me but the health visitor remained unconvinced. No further action was required but this experience gave the smallest of hints to the problems that lay ahead.

However, the first bombshell to rock the family was only months away and it would have nothing to do with doctors, medical problems or me.

Chapter Three
A Midnight Flit

I was only 18 months old when mum decided one night to pack her bags, grab her daughters and flee Skye, leaving Archie behind.

Over the years we've learned what happened to cause the break-up of their marriage, but to their credit both would simply say that they had their reasons. Neither wanted us to turn against the other, despite what may have gone on between them.

Islanders were intrigued by the midnight flit. Although, it was more of an evening escape, which left Archie gob-smacked as mum announced she was leaving and taking the kids. Knowing only that she would head for Dufftown, she hoped Rob would take us in. Everyone was stunned, including nana and grandpa and the rest of mum's family; all of whom were in the dark about what had prompted her to up sticks and bolt. Mum was determined not to let what went on between them pollute their relationship with Archie. After all, he was still practically living in, and running, the hotel with his in-laws.

Rob, nine years older than Margaret, did indeed take us in, but one thing was clear; if mum thought disappearing would be the end of the situation, she was wrong. Within days, Archie travelled to Dufftown with our aunt and uncle (mum's brother and sister-in-law) demanding the children return with him to Skye. We were all told to hide in the bathroom, with Rob's son Michael keeping guard, as our parents slugged it out on the doorstep. Frustrated with getting nowhere, Archie finally relented, spun on his heels and headed back over the sea to Skye. Not before, however, mum handed him the keys to the family car she had used to aid her flit. The fireworks would not end there though. Ten days later, when we believed things were quieting down and we were trying to adjust to life in Dufftown with Rob and Michael, Archie struck again. He arrived in the town with older brother Lachie, more in hope and desperation than expectation, and without a clear plan about what he would do. With luck, more than anything else, he spied Robina – her red Portree school uniform marking her out from her new classmates dressed in green – walking back to school after a lunch break. By then she was six and only enrolled in Primary Two in the local Mortlach Primary School. Seeing his opportunity, Archie pulled up alongside the startled youngster and, after he gestured her over to the car, Lachie hurriedly bundled her inside.

You might think such an ordeal would traumatise an impressionable young girl, but not Robina. She was thrilled. She thought being kidnapped was only the preserve of kids in the movies or Robert Louis Stevenson stories. Despite her only possessions being the clothes on her back, she was delighted to be with her dad and heading back to where her grandparents, friends and toys were. Plus, she got the day off school.

Mum, on the other hand, was furious. Yet swiftly she concluded that a messy custody battle over the children was not the way forward. Reluctantly, but showing a rather mature and innovative way of parenting, she agreed Robina would remain on Skye as long as she was happy, and Dorothy and I would join in her new life with Rob and Michael. She took comfort in the fact her parents and brothers were nearby, so Robina had access to the family for support. If Archie had decided to start a new life elsewhere, perhaps she would not have been so accommodating. However, Margaret knew she was regularly back in Skye and, although it broke her heart to be separated from her eldest child, she suppressed her own feelings and made do with the unorthodox situation for her daughter and the family's sake.

The compromise might have prevented full-scale warfare breaking out between the households but that did not mean it was a situation easy to live with. Although I was only a toddler when my parents separated, as I grew up the fact that Archie was my natural father became less of a concern for me. From an early age, I looked to Rob, as the man of the house, as my father figure. He was a wonderful dad and, right from the start, treated Dorothy and I as his own. But, while it was reasonably easy for me as a youngster to adjust to new situations, Dorothy was less able to make the transition smoothly. Putting myself in her shoes then, it must have been terribly confusing – her elder sister back home in Skye while she was left with the younger sibling hanging on her coat tails. How she must have yearned for her life back home because again, although young at the time of the split, she was old enough to have feelings about it and to understand what was happening.

My sister, then about to start school, probably had it the worst. Mum and Rob were alert to her sensitivity and tried everything they could to make her new life as happy as possible. Archie would phone the house every Sunday evening like clockwork, and at weekends and holidays she would be straight up to Skye to visit Robina and dad, if our eldest sister was not in Dufftown visiting us.

It was a difficult situation that could not have been easy for mum or Rob. There were so many dynamics in the house. Rob had his own concerns about his son Michael, much older than us girls, who was still coming to terms with the loss of his mother, and then having to deal with this ready-made family being shipped in en masse with our accompanying baggage. I am not going to pretend this unconventional set-up was a walk in the park and, as we grew older, we would all test the strength of our relationships to the limit, but we made it work. Thanks to their strength of character, mum, dad and Rob were able to make it happen for the kids.

Life in our new family moved on apace. Mum fell pregnant for a fourth time and she and Rob cemented their love for each other by tying the knot in Elgin Registry Office in September 1984, just a month after receiving the bit of paper which brought an end to her nine year marriage to Archie.

And there was more family joy when mum gave birth to another girl, Averil, eight weeks later and eighteen months after moving in with Rob. It looked touch and go with my little sister for a while when she was born. Weighing only four pounds at birth, she was breach and delivered four weeks early. She suffered breathing problems, requiring specialist attention. Thankfully, though, she made a full recovery and within days was home with us, fighting fit. I remember clearly her birth because Dorothy and I were decanted to stay with family friends, Averil and Leslie Aitken, who lived at the other end of the town. Their house was huge, with high ceilings and I remember Mrs Aitken put Dorothy and me in a room together with potties at the foot of each bed, even though we were six and three. Dot and I found it hilarious.

It was wonderful for mum and Rob to have a child together. They were obviously so in love and right for each other that it must have really seemed like it was making the family complete. At that time, we were living in a four-bedroom house in Conval Street, close to the town's famous clock tower. I shared a room with Dorothy, Michael had his own room and Averil slept in a cot in mum and Rob's en-suite master bedroom.

As we all adjusted to life with a new mouth to feed in the house, things were changing on Skye as well. Archie fell in love with local barmaid Shona and, while a few eyebrows were raised at the significant age gap (he was thirty-one, she was nineteen) they also married just a year later. Robina, by then nine, was delighted to have a female companion around the house and revelled in her new relationship with Shona who, because of the age gap, seemed more like a big sister than a step-mum.

So by the time I was four, I had a mum, a dad, a step-dad, a stepmother, a stepbrother and a half-sister. Archie and Shona would go on to have three children together, adding more half-siblings to the mix. But the technicalities are irrelevant. For the most part we were all one big happy family.

With Averil still a baby and me the closest to her in age, I would often remain in Dufftown with mum and Rob, while Dorothy was in Skye with Robina and Archie. If we did go west, more often than not I would stay with mum and everyone else at our grandparents' while Dorothy would stay at Archie's with Robina in the flat they were now living in at the back of the hotel. Like I said, we got on well together, for the most part.

Once, while I was staying at nana's but visiting Archie, Shona, Robina and Dorothy at the flat, I made sure my dad's new wife knew her place in the expanding brood. When she tried to scold me for misbehaving – which she was perfectly entitled to do in her own house of course – I ran into the kitchen, pulled a carving knife out of the drawer and brandished it at my dumb-struck stepmum.

"Who are you to tell me off?" I screamed. "You are not my mum."

Yes, things were a little confusing to say the least. Naturally I grew closer and fonder of Rob and began to call him dad. Averil was calling him dad, so why shouldn't I? On the times we did return to Skye as a family I would do the same, even in front of Archie and much to the annoyance of my big sisters who would tease me relentlessly for making dad shudder with sadness.

Robina had the best of both worlds, though. She still enjoyed her life in Skye with her friends and the rest of the family but she had her other life in Dufftown with us. I think one of the few times she felt sad about the split was when she had to select the toys which would be shipped on to Dorothy and I. Dorothy, probably envious of the life Robina had in Portree, was initially the one less accepting of Rob's role as dad to us all. She still kept in touch with Archie through regular phone calls, but my conversations with a man I saw to be a fairly distant relative many miles away grew less and less. Whenever I called Rob "dad", the pair of them would make me pay. They would say: "Why are you calling him dad? You've got a dad?"

Soon though, having decided the house they were living in was too small to accommodate a family of six, we moved into a purpose built house, just yards off Dufftown Main Street up a quiet private lane. The five-bedroom house, called Scorrybreck as a nod to the homestead on Skye, was to be our base pretty much until the present day.

After we moved in, we completed the family with a Springer Spaniel puppy called Ben. We all adored this little black and white ball of fluff. He grew into a crazy little mutt who would eat from a fork at the dinner table. He was the family pet but he took a particular shine to Averil and Michael, jumping on their beds when he was looking for a nap. It was all a bit crazy but it was the only family we knew and we just got on with it as best we could.

Sometimes it takes something quite significant to put the petty squabbles of every day life into perspective.

Chapter Four
Highland Flung

Eventually the storm subsided. Rob was working from home as an insurance agent. All the agents had their numbers and I recall he was number fourteen. The doorbell was forever ringing – morning, noon and even late at night – with clients calling to have their personal insurance problems sorted out for them. Once, a client even turned up at our door on Christmas Day to ask him to sort out their insurance claim. Rob just treated this selfishness as part and parcel of the job. He worked from an office at home and it was a great advantage having him around during the day but the drawback was that he also had to work evenings, doing his rounds. The same customers thought nothing of disturbing Rob, regardless of the hour but he was such an amiable chap and was happy to be of service.

The money from working such long hours was invaluable and soon we began to appreciate the comfortable standard of living afforded to us by Rob's hard work. It was a happy but hectic time. Just months after Averil's birth, mum opened a shop called M&Ms in the town square; selling women's and babies' clothes, with Rob's cousin Liz. Taking it in turns to run it, the two women juggled their roles as mums and housewives to make it work.

By the time I started at the local Mortlach Primary School as a four-year-old in 1985, no one could have begrudged mum for thinking that, after all the hurly-burly of recent years, she had finally found peaceful family life and something resembling a routine. Sadly, she would only feel such contentment briefly. There was no red-letter event to signify the underlying health problems her third daughter was suffering; only the little tell-tale signs that belied the trauma rumbling just beneath the surface of our happy existence.

Mum was the first to notice something was up. My first forays into school were nothing remarkable. I settled in reasonably well, made friends easily and, while I was no prodigy, did nothing of note to suggest Margaret had a problem

16

child on her hands. It wasn't until that terrible annual Sports Day, the social highlight of any primary school year, that mum started to suspect I was not like every other child on the field that day. She can remember looking puzzled as I struggled to keep up during the short sprint. As the other kids left me trailing in their wake, she realised it was not all connected to a lack of speed on my part. What seemed more likely was that I simply was not running like the other kids. Okay, she probably thought as I languished in last, 'She is not going to be Olympic sprint champion', but puzzlement became alarm as I hobbled along; my feet turned into each other and my back arched so much my head was angled up in the sky.

Looking along the row of mums excitedly cheering on from the sidelines, Margaret saw the expressions of joy and pride on their faces. Staring back at me, she tried to clap and smile like the rest, masking the inner fears that instinctively told her something was wrong with her daughter. Despite her concerns, there is surely no way she could have foreseen that this Primary One race would not be the last time my peers would leave me trailing. In reality, the warning signs had been there. As mum accompanied me on the short walk back to our house after the Sports Day, her mind began to replay the last few months of my life searching for any indication of a deeper meaning. As she started to think closely about my behaviour, mum realised she had noticed subtle problems with my co-ordination before.

There had been the situation at the highland dancing lessons for one thing. Dorothy and I had enrolled in the after-school class while I was still in Primary One. To the uninitiated, taking extra-curricular ceilidh lessons might sound extreme but to highlanders, dancing is a way of life. Many Scottish children owe their very existence to the passions raised by a vigorous night of country dancing. Maybe it is the bodies, swinging in close proximity, buoyed by gallons of drink, which loosens the inhibitions. So learning the steps to energetic jigs like the Dashing White Sergeant, the Eightsome Reel or the Gay Gordons is in many ways more vital to a child's sociological development than being able to master your Ps and Qs or knowing how to hold a knife and fork. In fact, for those who have never experienced a ceilidh before in their life, let me just

17

say that one dash through the hard-core spin fest which is Strip the Willow will make you ache in muscles you never knew you had.

And so, it was for our own physical fortitude and future ability to secure a mate, that mum sent Dorothy and I off to the afternoon dance fest. At first, I enjoyed the madness of it all. It was great fun being whirled around the room at great speeds and I could see no rhyme nor reason to the chaotic dance steps. I simply took it to be a freestyle dance-off, where you grabbed the nearest human being, preferably of the opposite sex, and tried to throw them over before they toppled you. Through the eyes of a five-year-old, it seemed that straightforward. That was until the teacher tapped me on the shoulder and gently whispered that in fact the jigs were carefully choreographed formation sequences. From then on, I may as well have tried to figure out the finer points of rocket science than get my head round the pas de basque and the many turns, circles, steps and waltzes.

Slowly I started to realise that the other children, including Dorothy, were able to pick up the intricacies of dance far quicker than me. Frustratingly, I realised there was no secret code to break, just the simple understanding that once you've been told how to do something for the twentieth time you should start to show improvement. Instead, I floundered and the more it seemed the teacher demanded I keep up and bellowed that I was holding up the entire class, the more pressure she heaped on top of me. Try as I might, I could not help but look foolish in front of my school chums. Despite my failings, it was still a surprise when the teacher asked my mum not to bring me to future classes. Mum was stunned that an instructor would mete such draconian punishment on a five-year-old girl.

It seems ridiculous now that a teacher would behave in such a manner. This was not a grooming camp for the Bolshoi ballet; it was after-school highland dancing in a town with a thousand people. Surely, adults should allow kids to be rubbish. Taking part is what counts. Obviously, this was not so in my case.

Mum could do nothing and she simply put it down to the assumption that highland dancing was not my forte. Naturally, she probably wondered what my true calling would be.

Margaret had passed that episode off as the ravings of an intolerant coach but now she was not so sure.

Soon, I started to develop other behavioural quirks. Simple tasks, like putting on shoes and socks and tying laces, became Herculean trials. I began to trip over my own feet and before long turned clumsiness into an art form. My sisters took great glee in taking the Mickey about my gait that rapidly resembled my peculiar running style. One leg would be straight but the other would be practically at right angles to it, with my left foot pointed inwards. They teased me for sitting awkwardly on the floor and giggled as I invariably lost my balance and tumbled over.

As any mother would, Margaret took me along to the local doctor for a check-up. Our family doctor was a kind, good-hearted man called Thomas Heneghan, whose practice has been caring for the people of Dufftown since long before we moved to the town. I would grow to know the waiting room inside out and give every one of the battered old toys the once over at some point. It was a small room, with about fifteen seats. The main feature was a glass aquarium on a table by the wall. If I was to count the total minutes I had spent in his practice, staring at the fish, I'm sure it would stretch into hours. This time, however, he gave me the once over but there was nothing to suggest I was anything other than a clumsy little girl still getting used to her body and perhaps a little behind my classmates physically. Surely, this was not normal behaviour for a child my age, mum queried. The doctor assured her it was. Mum was not convinced. She demanded further tests but the doctor was at a loss what to test for. My vital signs were fine and there were no indications of an underlying problem.

As quickly as the first signs appeared, now more symptoms were following in their wake. I started to complain of dull headaches seeming to throb from the centre of my skull. I became restless at night and struggled to sleep for long periods. The tiredness sapped my energy levels and my eyesight started to flag. Soon my vision began to blur as I felt my body start to slow down.

Mum was not the only one in the family to notice differences between me and other children. Once, on Skye, while we were at the Portree swimming pool with Shona, she noticed a strange, glazed expression in my eyes, as if I was not able to focus clearly on the activity around me. As the other children splashed and had fun, I sat trapped in my own world. Then one morning Dorothy woke me from a drowsy slumber to find my head stuck to the pillow. As she peeled aside my hair, she noticed thick, yellowy goo on the side of my face. By the time I woke up, I was horrified to see the entire right side of my face covered in the waxy substance, seemingly coming from my ear. Rob and my mum were also shocked and hastily arranged another check-up with the doctor, who by now was becoming more and more used to our visits.

In August of that year, mum had me back at the doctor. She was now highly agitated and had catalogued a host of problems in my behaviour. My legs were constantly stiff, I was tired and sleepy all the time; even through the school holidays at the end of Primary One, when children are meant to be energised. The latent squint, spotted when I was a year old, seemed to have returned but only presented itself now and then. The headaches I had been complaining of had become more frequent and I had begun to drink excessively, seemingly never able to quench my thirst.

Dr Heneghan sympathised with mum's anxieties. He decided to refer me to a specialist at Aberdeen Royal Infirmary. He believed my walking co-ordination problems stemmed from a muscle problem in my legs, but looking into my eyes he could also tell there was a build of pressure behind the pupils.

Eyes may be the windows of the soul but medics know they can also provide a view into the brain as well. The eye is the only part of the human anatomy where you can actually see a nerve at work – the optic nerve. A redness of the blood vessels and the paleness of the nerve itself, seen during an examination, can be an indicator of pressure on the veins. The eye reacts in the same way your leg would if you tied a garter extremely tight – eventually it leads to swelling of the foot.

When the doctor looked into my eyes, he detected a swelling round the edge that normally would have been crisp and flat. Often with raised pressure in the veins to the nerve, doctors can detect a papilledema (swelling in the optic disc and veins), a common sign in sufferers of multiple sclerosis and a telltale sign of pressure on the brain. When Dr Heneghan spotted these symptoms, he knew it was time to refer me to specialists in Aberdeen. He made an appointment for me to go through to the Granite City to try to find the source of my problems. I never made it to that appointment. Not long after the meeting was set, events were to overtake themselves as my condition rapidly deteriorated.

It was an afternoon like any other, with Michael, Dorothy, mum and I in the house preparing for dinner. Rob was out on his rounds, seeing clients around Dufftown. I got up and made my way from the lounge through the hallway to the dining-kitchen area on the same level to get a glass of juice. It was hardly scaling the north face of the Eiger. However, it was beyond me. Without warning, I crashed headlong into the edge of the kitchen doorframe and, before I knew it, lay pole-axed on the floor. Mum panicked and sent Michael and Dorothy out to find Rob. These were the days before mobile phones and he could have been in the house of any one of his regular customers. Dorothy and Michael split up and, while mum tried to bring me round in the house, they raced round his clients, going door-to-door searching for him. Michael eventually found him and brought him back to the house immediately. In the mayhem, no one could find poor Dorothy to tell her, and – bless her – she stalked the streets for an hour, despite being just eight-years-old.

Mum rushed me back to the doctor in the morning where he agreed a hastier appointment. However, that afternoon, taking matters into my own hands again, I collapsed at the fence at the front of the house. Mum gasped, fearing her little girl was slipping away. It was a momentary black out and I soon regained consciousness and composure, but I was quickly on my way to Aberdeen Royal Infirmary. I didn't know it then, but the place would become my home for the next five years.

Chapter Five
Under Pressure

I have to rely on my family to tell me the specifics of my first visit to Aberdeen Royal Infirmary because by the time doctors admitted me my condition had deteriorated quite markedly. From simply showing a few signs of clumsiness just weeks before, I was now reeling from the same kind of symptoms I would rediscover some 15 years later. The pressure on my brain was now unbearable and excruciatingly throbbed through my skull. The veins on my head started to swell and instinctively I found it harder and harder to raise my head up. My eyes shied away from bright light and those things I could see began to blur and merge.

It must have been terrifying for mum and Rob who were naturally alarmed at the speed at which I was deteriorating. The drive through from Dufftown to Aberdeen must have taken forever. They prayed that the specialists would have the answer to my problems and watched as their child seemed to be gradually, but swiftly, shutting down.

It was to the town's Royal Infirmary, where the renowned neurology department serves patients from the entire north of Scotland, that specialists summoned mum and Rob to take me for my first CT scan. Awaiting the results of that scan must have been torture for them both. On one hand, they were desperate to know what was taking over their daughter, while on the other, dreading what the doctors would tell them. The scan showed a mass of grey fluid building up on my brain, possibly the same goo Dorothy had spotted on my pillow. The experts mentioned some of the common causes of fluid build-up on the brain, including tumours, but they were unclear what the root of my problem was. As far as they knew, my condition could have stemmed from a blockage at birth that only recently had decided to present itself. One thing they did agree on was that the situation called for immediate action.

It was hydrocephalus. To any normal family the word has no meaning whatsoever. The specialists explained the name was

Greek (its translation literally meaning water on the brain) but, as doctors talked them through what the diagnosis meant for their daughter; they might as well have been speaking in a foreign language for all the sense the technical jargon made. For mum, only the main points hammered home. There was a blockage on the brain. It had caused a build up of fluid. The pressure was growing on my skull. They would need to operate right away. By this time, consultants had admitted me to the children's ward near the main building. When surgeons diagnose hydrocephalus they want to act right away and to delay action is to speed up death.

My head, now swollen severely over my eyes, looked as though the smallest pin would burst it like a water balloon. My legs lay rigid and stiff as wooden logs. Mum squeezed my hand but I could not see her even though she sat just inches away from my face. I was effectively blind. The pain in my head was now so great I couldn't have opened my eyes even if I'd wanted to. Mum and Rob sat by my bedside, terrified at what the next few hours might bring. They watched, horrified, as doctors tried desperately to take a blood sample in preparation for surgery. My veins had collapsed and repeatedly doctors stabbed into my body in a futile attempt to find a vessel to give up some blood.

Until that point, I had been drifting in and out of consciousness but now I was screaming in pain, hysterical as still the medics battled for a blood sample. First, they tried my arms, then legs before finally prizing a trickle from my foot. As I writhed in agony, mum feared the surgery would be too late, that angels would take me before the surgeons had sterilised their hands. At one point, seeing me in so much agony, she even wished for it to end there. Certain there was no way out of this living hell, she prayed that if I did make it under the surgeon's knife, I would never wake up from the anaesthetic. Surely, that would at least mean a peaceful end rather than prolonging my torture.

Finally, the ordeal was over and it was time to kiss me goodnight for the last time before surgery the following morning. Rob held mum as they walked out of the ward. The two of them stayed overnight in the hospital's Craig Unit, a dedicated facility for parents of sick children just down the corridor from Ward Four, where they would be able to sleep. Furnished with a handful of bedrooms and a communal kitchen, it was a Godsend for people like us, who were travelling from outside the area. As Aberdeen serviced the whole of the north-east of Scotland, many parents were grateful for the chance to stay close to their loved ones in their time of need.

In the lift, they met the neurosurgeon, David Currie. He informed mum that he would be operating on me in the morning. Mum looked him straight in the eye and pleaded, "Operate as if it is your own daughter." He promised he would do everything in his power to save her little girl.

The following morning mum and Rob were back at my bedside and walked with me as I went for the anaesthetic. They waved me off into the operating theatre but, as the doors closed, mum wondered if it would be the last time she would see me alive. Before the operation, I had no idea what was going on because I was too ill; no idea what was causing me so much pain or what would happen to me to make it better. However, the consultants talked mum through the situation and the risks major surgery could have on the brain of a five-year-old girl.

Of course, as is often the case with medical terminology, the phrase "water on the brain" only tells part of the story. To give you a crash course in the inner workings of the head, the water is in fact cerebrospinal fluid, a clear liquid that fills the ventricles of the brain, passing through to the stem before flowing to the top surface of the skull and down to the spinal chord. It assists the body's central nervous system and protects the soft tissue inside the head from sudden knocks and jarring movements. Normally this fluid should drain away into the bloodstream through large veins but if they block in any way the fluid builds up, causing the head to swell, putting pressure on the eyes and, take it from me, causing headaches on a grand scale. Often brain diseases like meningitis or haemorrhages stop the fluid flowing normally and cause communicating hydro-cephalus. However, most commonly, blockages from foreign bodies lead to the build up of pressure.

In my case, surgeons could not see an obvious cause for the logjam so put my condition down to communicating hydro-cephalus.

If I had been born thirty years previously, the chances are I would not have seen my sixth birthday. In the 1950s, children diagnosed with the condition stood only a 15% chance of survival. Those who did usually stayed permanently in hospital, retarded and blind, living out their lives with tubes draining excess fluid from their grotesquely large heads. That changed with the birth of Casey Holter, an American boy born in November 1955 with a severe form of spina bifida. As if that was not enough for his anguished parents to contend with, he contracted meningitis shortly after birth, causing his head to expand rapidly. Next, his doctors confirmed he had hydrocephalus. Fortunately, if luck ever smiled on such a tragic family, Casey was being treated at the same Philadelphia hospital where neurosurgeons Eugene Spitz and Frank Nulsen had discovered a drainage system from the brain to the stomach that might work. What they needed was a valve to control the direction of the flow that would stop the heat pumping fluid drained from the brain back into the head. Casey's death sentence devastated his father John Holter, an engineer for the Yale and Town Lock Company, who strived to overcome what he saw as a relatively simple plumbing problem. He devised a silicone valve that operated one way, allowing the fluid to flow away from the brain but prevented it returning. He developed the first shunt and carried out the testing on his own boy. Miraculously, it was successful for a while but, as is still often the case with hydrocephalus, Casey needed replacements soon afterwards and, tragically, died from an epileptic fit at the tender age of five.

However, word soon spread about the Holter miracle shunt as neurosurgeons across America began to hear about the breakthrough. There was a desire to push ahead with the new technology because patients were living death sentences without it. Scientists added rubber to the silicone to make a medically suitable substance Silastic – now also used in breast implants and heart valves – and the Spitz-Holter shunt was born. Although Casey lost his brave battle for life, fifty years later the device has turned the figures on their head and, thanks to his remarkable father, children now born with hydrocephalus stand an 85% chance of living a long and happy life.

Another child to benefit from the Spitz-Holter valve was Theo Dahl, son of best-selling children's author, Roald Dahl. However, when the valve kept blocking as a result of bleeding in the brain, Roald set about devising a new valve with an engineer friend, Stanley Wade. They added two metal discs to help prevent future blockages.

Today there are more than 40 valves in use but it is to the Spitz-Holter design I owe my life. Fitting a shunt in 1987 was a standard procedure but try telling my mum that as she watched medics wheel me into the operating theatre. Once they bore into the back of your head, surgeons fit the shunt in three parts – the valve was fixed behind the ear at the side of the neck with a wire attached running down the body and anchored in the peritoneal cavity in the abdomen; a space there where fluid could be absorbed. It was fitted with a coiled wire so there was less chance of the tube kinking.

I don't know if mum kept hearing the words "standard procedure" echoing round her head during the time I was under the surgeon's knife, but those words must have sounded more and more hollow, the longer I took to emerge. She was pacing up and down the wards near to the recovery area. Rob kept telling her to calm down, that I was in the hands of the experts and that everything would be okay. However, as the clock ticked on, her maternal instinct told her she could not be so sure. The time Mr Currie had said for the operation had come and gone but, as Margaret looked vainly for someone to put her out of her misery, no one could give her the answer she was looking for.

She grew more and more agitated as minutes became hours and still there was no word from the operating theatre. Eventually, some two hours after the scheduled end of the operation, a nurse spoke to my mum. There was good news and bad news. Obviously, a healthcare professional would not put it as flippantly as that but mum was in no doubt what she was telling her. The good news was I was out of theatre and the operation had appeared to be a success. The bad news was they were struggling to revive me.

Mum, too upset and scared to call her parents directly, called my uncle with the latest news. He arrived at the hospital with my nana and grandpa. Mum was distressed. Her dad had been struggling recently with heart problems and she was worried what the sight of his granddaughter so sick in hospital might do to him. Yet they arrived as the nurses continued to try waking me from the anaesthetic. My grandparents watched with dismay and horror as nurses pinched my ear and tried any other sharp shock tactics to revive me.

Finally, it took a nurse digging her nail right into my ear to effect a response from this five-year-old girl. When at last I came to, I was barely conscious. Sick from the anaesthetic, I could not even lift my head to vomit. I still could not see, my legs felt like ten tonne weights and the pain in my head had only marginally subsided.

For nana and grandpa it was terrible. How awful to see their granddaughter gravely ill in hospital and their own daughter so upset and powerless to help. Mum was beside herself with worry but, struggling to keep a lid on her emotions, she tried desperately to shield her anguish from her parents.

Tragically, it was just too much for grandpa. His heart could not take it and he took a turn right there in the ward. He collapsed, short of breath, clutching his chest. Everyone gasped, believing the unthinkable was happening in front of their eyes. The ward, designed for recovery and with an atmosphere of recuperation and stability, suddenly turned into a hotbed of activity as nurses jumped to deal with the emergency.

Thankfully, grandpa's condition – while extremely serious – stabilised but he still required treatment.

Therefore, as if dealing with my situation wasn't enough, mum had to watch as two ambulances came for two members of her family; one to take grandpa to the main casualty department of the infirmary and another to ferry me from the recovery ward to the nearby sick children's hospital on the same campus.

The following morning mum had to divide her time between her dad and daughter. We were both in wheelchairs in opposite ends of the hospital complex. At least for my part, I had picked up a little. Although I could sit up, I was still very poorly and felt sick from the effects of the anaesthetic.

While it might not have been obvious at the time, the operation had been a success. The shunt was already doing its job, working through the excess fluid built up on my brain. However, like a blocked sink, it was going to take a while for the blockage to clear and, before it did, the symptoms were ever present. Yet, as each day passed following the operation, I became a little stronger and gradually my personality started to show itself again.

As I recovered in a cubicle in Ward Four of the children's hospital, I was delighted my uncle was there. He had always had a soft spot for me and I enjoyed the banter we had together. Soon I was showing off my scar to him, which was quite impressive – stretching from the back of my head to the bottom of my neck. My only concern was that they had chopped off my cherished long brown hair before the operation to allow the surgeon to do his work. For a young girl that really is a matter of life and death.

Chapter Six
Hydro What?

The neurosurgeon, Mr Currie, kept his promise to mum. He had operated as if it was his own daughter lying in front of him.

As my senses returned, I began to grasp what had happened to me. I had no idea before the operation of the seriousness of the situation facing me, nor the drama that unfolded in the hospital.

Due to my delirious state, it was felt unwise to try to explain the intricacies of what was about to happen. However, after the emergency had passed, the surgeons considered me well enough to know what was going on inside my body. With mum at my side, the specialists explained the hydrocephalus and the impact it had on my wellbeing. They talked me through my operation, describing in detail the procedure and how I was now different from many girls and boys my age. The concept that a man-made drainage system in my brain was keeping me alive was a difficult one to comprehend. Even now, I am not entirely sure I fully appreciate how lucky I am. Yet, according to mum and the surgeons, I seemed to take in what they were saying. Certainly, given the amount of time I was to spend in the sick children's hospital following the surgery, I had plenty of time to contemplate my situation.

Although I had a rather attractive bandage covering most of the back of my head, I could feel the shunt under my skin at the right hand side of my neck. Despite being small and fragile, the tube felt like any old pipe running down the side of my head. Probably because the only thing I could picture in my mind to relate to the device was a rubber hose, I imagined something like that was winding its way through my body to my stomach like an overflow pipe. It was weird to think someone had gone inside my head and fiddled around, in the same way Rob would tinker about under the bonnet of his car. In fact, the surgeon had opened me up three times, in the head, collarbone and stomach and, morbidly, I imagined what it must have been like. I suppose it was just my way of coming to terms with major brain surgery.

I was a long time in hospital following the operation. Rehabilitation was a slow process. Essentially, doctors said I would have to learn to walk all over again. The consultants warned mum there was a danger of paralysis with the operation – as there is any time surgeons go fiddling about inside the brain – and her fear was that there would be some serious lasting damage from the surgery. An intensive programme of physiotherapy began with simple exercises to get my joints moving again. It had seemed so long since I last used them in earnest that it felt like Mr Currie had chopped them off during surgery.

The pressure eased on my brain and slowly the swelling started to subside above my eyes. Gradually I was able to lift my eyes towards light, but it was to remain several weeks until my eyesight returned to its previous sharpness.

When I first woke up, my speech was slurred. To me I sounded fine, as the words sounded crystal clear in my own head, but mum was alarmed to hear me sound like a stroke victim. However the speech, like my sight, slowly came back as the pressure eased on my brain.

Considering I was still just a five-year-old girl, I grew used to being in hospital and became quite accustomed to life on the children's ward. For one thing, the amount of presents I received far outstripped my wildest imagination. As you can imagine all our friends and family were extremely worried and, after the operation, that concern manifested itself in dolls, toys and games.

The Royal Aberdeen Children's Hospital sits five hundred yards from the main Foresterhill site of the city's infirmary. The building, on one level, catered for all paediatric needs. The ward I was always admitted to was Ward Four, set aside for the most serious cases – cancers, leukaemia, brain tumours and meningitis. There were about twenty beds on one side for the older kids, while the other side was taken up with cribs for the tiniest of babies. At night time, the nurses switched lights off at 9pm, yet, despite the number of children on the ward, it was a peaceful place to be. The nurses themselves were kind and always maintained a cheery atmosphere on the wards, in spite of the trauma they must have faced on a daily basis. Seeing children succumb to the most terrible of illnesses must have been heartbreaking for them, especially with the bond they built up with the kids on the ward.

Shortly after the surgery, mum and Rob agreed that, as his work demanded he was back in Dufftown, he would return home while she remained in Aberdeen with me. The hospital provided accommodation for parents of sick kids and mum was able to sleep overnight in a room not far from me. On the occasions she returned home, she arrived back laden with more gifts from well-wishers. The other girls in my family could not believe it. For them, my stay in hospital was a curiosity. Mum and Rob explained to them the seriousness of the situation but, sparing them the gory details of the surgery, emphasised the positive aspects and assured them I would soon be back home as normal. Therefore, as it was, they enjoyed coming through to Aberdeen to visit for different reasons. Dorothy and Michael loved racing each other up and down the corridors on vacant wheelchairs and seemed to spend more time busying themselves with the available toys than spending hours holding my hand by my bedside.

I have to admit I never gave the fact that mum was with me throughout my stay a second thought. I had never had to do without her before that point so it was natural, and comforting to have her there. In addition, for mum, there was never any question of her being anywhere else. However, it is only now I appreciate the sacrifice she made with regard to the other children. Averil was just two when my illness showed itself and mum must have felt terribly divided between being there for her sick child and fulfilling her role at home. I suppose, once the operation was out the way, mum might have been forgiven for believing once I'd recovered I could expect to lead a reasonably normal life but her devotion to my situation started in earnest in hospital that time.

Very soon, however, she was going to get a taste of just how demanding hydrocephalus is – and how patients rely on vigilant medics for their very survival.

As I slowly regained my strength, the doctors were mindful of other possible complications regarding the shunt. The device can be prone to infection, causing serious problems, and blockages were still an ever-present worry. Surgeons told my worried parents they would have to monitor the shunt for the rest of my life because an unchecked build-up of pressure on my brain could kill me. Another irregularity was my height. For months doctors had been closely monitoring my physical development. After a healthy start in life, I had fallen behind the average height for kids my age. Following the surgery, the consultants warned mum and Rob I might not reach full height. It was yet another factor they would keep a close eye on. The doctors also recommended I go for another CT scan. The surgeons were still keen to find a possible source of the blockage and even checked for signs of a spinal tumour. No clue was forthcoming but they did notice the build up of fluid on my brain had returned.

Therefore, just one month after the original operation, I was back in the operating theatre, this time under the supervision of neurosurgeon Christopher Blaiklock. The shunt had blocked. Initially, the first valve had worked well releasing the build-up of fluid but latterly the excess water had proved too much for the shunt and Mr Blaiklock decided to revise the device. The operation was far more straightforward the second time round and, as I had already been recovering, I made far better progress following surgery.

Soon the time came for me to return home, some two months after I'd first been admitted. Having missed the start to my second year at primary school it was difficult at first to readjust to school life. My boyish haircut still caused me palpitations and I was conscious of the attention my bandage and bald patch would attract at school. After all, not many children in class could list having undergone life-saving brain surgery under their holiday news when returning for their second year after the summer break!

My first morning back was particularly chilly so mum decided it best to drive me the few yards to the school gates. A small gesture, but it was preferential treatment like that which was to have a significant impact on my behaviour in later years.

In class, I got the first inclination that I was different from most children and that people might treat me differently when my teacher, Mrs Winifred McWilliam said kindly to me after a lesson; "I've popped a sweetie into your satchel." Other aspects of my schooling only added to this belief. Although surgeons stressed with mum that the shunt would not hinder my life in any great way, gym or sport was now off the curriculum. For that, I was grateful, as I had never shown any special talent for physical activity. However, my condition did have its implications. I exhausted very easily and grew reliant on afternoon naps to help me through the day. So, for the first few weeks at school I could only manage half days. My eyesight had failed to recover to a degree acceptable for reading and writing and my GP recommended I see an optician. He confirmed I was short sighted and so I began my life-long dependency on glasses and I returned to school with spectacles that would have embarrassed even Elton John.

Suddenly I was getting a crash course in how to deal with a serious health problem. As I was sent to bed in the afternoon, I started to rebel. I could not understand the full implications of what was wrong with me and I could not see why I had to go to bed while other children were at school. As I lay there in bed, I hated hearing the noises of the outside world beyond my curtains. Although tired, this was not like I had experienced in hospital, where going to bed whenever you felt like forty winks was the norm. Here I felt I was missing out. I would sit up in bed and peek out the blinds to see what was going on. Little did I know it but my behaviour then was the first inclination that I would develop a rebellious streak in retaliation to the constraints my condition would put on my life.

In reality, Primary Two was a washout for me at school. Starting my education at four, I had been one of the youngest in my class but had been able to keep up with the older chums during the early days. However, missing a huge chunk of the school year put me under a lot of pressure to keep up. While I had been in hospital, Dorothy had tried to keep mum up to date with school work I was missing and the sick kids hospital ran a makeshift classroom setting to ensure patients did not miss out too much on their schoolwork, but it wasn't the same as being

33

in the disciplined environment of a class setting. If you add to that my inability to last a full day, it soon became clear I would not progress like other children my age.

With the specialists in Aberdeen now keen to keep a regular check on the effectiveness of my new shunt and continue their hunt for the source of the blockage, they sent me for six monthly CT scans to monitor my progress.

In 1987, such images, known as computerised topography, or CAT scans were commonplace in hospitals. Devised by Sir Godfrey Hounsfield, who went on to win the Nobel Prize for his innovation, the advantage of CT over an x-ray was that, rather than taking a one-dimensional silhouette of the skull, the scan could show up much more detail. Hounsfield devised a machine that, instead of showing a silhouette of the body, fired a beam of x-rays attached to a gantry. As the beam went through the body, the gantry moved the length, with the beam adjusting a degree each time to map the skull using the data provided from the images. A computer uses this information to work out the relative density of the tissues examined. Each set of measurements made by the scanner is a cross-section through the body. The computer processes the results, displaying them as a two-dimensional picture shown on a monitor.

The first hospital in the UK to receive such a scanner was the Atkinson Morley hospital in Wimbledon where, lucky enough for me, a young Mr Blaiklock also happened to be.

When Hounsfield initially invented the machine, it took nine days to compile the results. Thankfully, by the time I was ready to use it, the results arrived much quicker. Getting the first scan was a strange experience, lying like a corpse on a mortuary slab was unnerving as the beams penetrated my body. However, by the time I had my third scan, shortly after the second operation, I felt I was an old hand at the procedure and started to look forward to entering the machine that moved me forwards and backwards while it snapped every inch of my brain. It was a good job I did not mind the process because the scanners were to feature prominently in my life in the years to come.

At the same time, I was frequently at my local doctor for regular check-ups. Like many patients who have a history of brain problems, I was now accustomed to the rather unorthodox tests carried out to detect underlying neurological issues. One such test is the planter reflex, demonstrated by the doctor scraping the sole of the foot from heel to toe. This causes the big toe to bend down the way. If the toe bends up the way then it is a sign of possible problems in the brain. If not then it could be an indication of something more serious. Another response they checked me for was how my muscles reacted to stretching. The way to test this is by sharply bending up the foot at the ankle to trigger the response. A rhythmic jerking to this manoeuvre might again suggest deep-rooted neurological problems. To add to this, the paediatrician measured the circumference of my head for more swelling and regularly demanded I run, hop, skip and jump so he could check my vital neurological signs.

In the months following the shunt operations, nothing in my development gave great cause for concern in the eyes of experts. One aspect of good news was that I had enjoyed my first growth spurt in a year. It looked like I wasn't going to remain a Munchkin after all. However, constant tiredness and a failure to shake off the throbbing headaches meant that, in my mind at least, I could never be satisfied that my worst days were behind me.

Chapter Seven
Two Carolines

The months that followed brought mixed emotions. For the most part the shunt, since the revision, had been doing its job. The swelling above my eyes had subsided and perhaps the doctors were right; the build up of pressure which almost cost me my life had indeed been caused by a blockage in my brain since birth. None of the neurological tests displayed anything other than symptoms commonly associated with hydrocephalus.

Despite this, I still had the niggling suspicion of something being not quite right. I had been in a state of discomfort for so long now it was hard to remember what normality was like. I was still suffering from headaches but my consultant assured my mum this was still an after-effect of the hydrocephalus and a condition that I would have to learn to live with. My awkward gait, the tell-tale sign that had first set alarm bells ringing, was a symptom surgery couldn't fix. Forced to wear clumpy, old-fashioned shoes to rectify my disobedient legs, I cursed mum, as if it was her fault, for making me look foolish. Although having just turned six and owing my life to our health professionals, I still wasn't going to be told what was good for me; especially if it was at the sacrifice of fashion. I felt the shoes only served to draw attention to my clumsy legs.

To be fair, my local GP, Dr Tom Heneghan, and the paediatricians at Aberdeen, were always encouraging me to live as normal a life as possible. Yet, owing to the surgery, there were always going to be limitations. My tolerance levels for strenuous physical activity were never going to put Liz McColgan to shame but now, following my surgery, I ran out of puff quicker than a forty-a-day smoker. But the message was clear – this was to be my normality and the sooner I accepted it the better.

Remarkably, things did improve for a while. Encouraged by mum and envious of the fun Dorothy seemed to have in the uniform, I joined the Brownies. This was great fun and for the first time in a long time enabled me to feel like one of the girls.

Sure, I couldn't keep up with them on the sporting activities and I used to get in a tangle with my lopsided co-ordination but, dressed in the brown dress and yellow neckerchief, I forgot about what was going on inside my brain. My ongoing health problems had rendered it almost impossible for me to take part in after-school activities and I had lost interest in hobbies, so I liked the social nature of the sausage sizzles, campfires and walks.

I also enrolled in the school choir, much to the delight of mum who loved seeing her children participating in community activities. She had given up the shop because she had wanted to devote her attention to me, one of several sacrifices she had to make for me. Again, being part of an ensemble whisked me away from my trials, if only momentarily. I loved that. I have always considered myself to be the best singer ever and I am convinced a pop career would have beckoned were it not for my problems!

However, if I was starting to think I had the measure of the hydrocephalus, something else was thrown into the mix to put all of my frustrations regarding the shunt and the limitations it put on my life, into the shade. In many ways the deterioration in my health came on just like the water on the brain. The headaches I'd become accustomed to increased in frequency and ferocity. To the uninitiated it's hard to describe these headaches, but imagine someone had climbed inside your skull and was bashing your brain with a hammer and you're close. School became an alien concept for me as day after day I was crippled by such punishing migraines. The tiredness, which by now was my trademark, scaled new heights, rendering me useless for most of the day and, as if that wasn't enough to contend with, I discovered a shooting pain in my abdomen to accompany the throbbing sensation in my skull.

Over the coming months I was such a regular at Dr Heneghan's practice that mum should have had her own parking space. Yet again the symptoms were dismissed as a reaction to the hydrocephalus, perhaps related to the fact I was growing. In the house, I grew irritated at the slightest commotion and grumpy at loud noises, which in a house with four kids meant practically all the time. My parents tried to reassure me about my recurring health problems but surely inside they knew that any hope they may have had that the worst was over was only wishful thinking.

In the days I did manage to get to school, I required remedial assistance to try and keep up with my classmates but at that age it was a futile exercise. Losing over a year of schooling would be a tall order for any youngster, never mind one riddled with health problems.

My situation only strengthened mum's resolve to treat me like the other kids and I was required to accompany the other girls on trips to the swimming pool. However the intoxicating smell of chlorine and the unnaturally warm atmosphere of the baths only served to further intensify my headaches. My legs grew stiff again and I found walking as tricky as maths lessons in school. Without explanation I started walking on my tiptoes and moved along in jerky, spiky steps. Any hopes of a recall to the highland dancing were most definitely out of the question now.

I continued to undergo CT scans on my head to assess my progress but the specialists often found the results as confusing as the explanations for my bizarre behaviour. My consultants, desperate to find the root of the problems, were often left frustrated by the scans because the stem, a crucial area of my brain, was difficult to analyse properly in the scans. Yet still they persisted and, in October 1990, two months from my ninth birthday I was summoned for another. Waiting for the results of the scans is even worse than knowing the answers they reveal, mum used to say. She hated the endless hanging about in hospitals. Sometimes we would travel back to Dufftown from Aberdeen after the procedure or, alternatively, we would wait in the hospital for the results. At times it felt like they were using Sir Godfrey Hounsfield's original prototype scanner that took nine days to give up its secrets. This was one of those times.

With me in the children's ward (ward four) of the nearby sick kid's hospital was Caroline Nicol, a pretty blonde girl born six months before me, and who lived just twenty miles away in Elgin. Caroline and her parents, Liz and Vince, were familiar faces in a ward where misery lorded over happiness. It always baffled mum how a room so full of children could ever have an atmosphere so laden with sorrow. She used to look round the room with tears in her eyes at the tragic faces staring back. So many young lives blighted. Some children had leukaemia, others recovering from meningitis. One boy had a tumour on his face. Yet, to see the way some of these brave kids walked around the ward, it was clear no one had told them they were the unlucky ones.

And then there was Caroline. When our families first met, Caroline's bed was at the opposite end of the ward from mine. She was a very pretty little girl and good fun. Mum and Rob hit it off immediately with Liz and Vince. We marvelled at the similarities in our situations, despite the terrible circumstances which had brought us together. Our names were almost identical. At the time, I technically still carried Archie's family moniker Nicolson. Only six months separated us and yet we had both been diagnosed with hydrocephalus and each had shunts fitted in our heads. It was remarkable how many things we shared. We grew close in the wards and I always looked forward to seeing her, even though sadly, our meetings meant we were both still plagued by our afflictions.

On the day we were awaiting the results of my scan, Caroline was there too, also for a scan. She was very poorly. Her shunt, fitted only months previously, seemed to have blocked and it looked like surgeons would have to operate again, much like they did with me. We had been talking that day. Caroline and I played with toys on the ward, while the parents yakked. Mum and Liz had grown close in the brief time they had known one another, sharing the same wicked sense of humour to get them through these troubling times. It was the day before Halloween and, like we did, the Nicols faced an agonising wait for their results. It was 5.50pm when the consultant paediatrician finally entered the room. Parents rose expectantly, hoping it would be their turn to be put out of their misery first. This time though, it was Caroline who was at the head of the queue. The consultant beckoned Liz and Vince to the small room at the side of the ward. They seemed to be in there for an eternity. In reality it was barely 10 minutes. Her mum and dad left the room looking as though they had seen a ghost. We were next to see the consultant. Mum had a brief moment to quickly ask Liz what had happened. "It's a tumour," she said. Mum was shaking. Good God, no. Then it was mum and Rob's turn to be summoned into the visitor's room. But, as they sat down, mum's thoughts were with the Nicols. Surely though, she thought, that has to be the bad news for the day?

The tiny, enclosed space only comprised of a table, some chairs, a jug of water and a box of tissues; all the requirements for a piece of bad news. The consultant was blunt. The latest CT scan showed a tumour sitting in the middle of my brain. It measured 1.5 centimetres, less than the diameter of a 1p coin. Mum stared in disbelief.

"It can't be," she gasped. "You have made a mistake. Check again. You've got the wrong Caroline. It's Caroline Nicol who has the tumour. We're Caroline Nicolson. There's been a mix up. I've just spoken to her parents."

She probably said out loud what her mind wanted her to hear. Surely two girls called Caroline couldn't be diagnosed with tumours on the same day? The consultant had been expecting such a reaction. "We double-checked when we saw the similarities. I'm sorry, but there is no mistake."

Mum was incredulous. So many questions. What did this mean? Was it cancerous? Could they operate? It was a low-grade pineal tumour. It was sitting in the centre of my brain. The consultant said it was less cancerous than some tumours, but its mere presence on the brain gave cause for serious concern.

Then, while mum and Rob were on the ropes with that news, came the sucker punch: it was inoperable. I was stuck with this ticking time-bomb in my head. Mr Blaiklock had looked at the scan but could not find a way in. Their advice was simple: take me home and try and enjoy Christmas together, the inference being it would be our last as a family. I was eight, just about to turn nine. It was highly unlikely I would see ten.

When mum and Rob came out of the room, I was oblivious to what was going on. I had been sitting on the bed by the toilet door in the ward while my parents were getting the news that would send the bottom crashing out of their world. Mum came over and hugged me tightly. We sat talking for a bit but neither of them gave anything away as to the seriousness of the situation. Yet the longer mum spent in the ward the more agitated she became. Mum explained she was leaving me overnight in the hospital. She was going back to Dufftown. She could not bear to be in that hospital any longer. She was going to go back home and would return first thing in the morning. I thought it was strange. I didn't mind, but mum had never left me alone overnight in the hospital before. She normally slept in the parents' room nearby.

That night, mum and Rob never slept a wink. Mum kept replaying the conversation with the consultant over and over again. Something must be done, she thought. There has to be something they can do.

The following morning, mum showed no signs of the heartache ripping her apart inside. I was already up and dressed when I saw them come in through the ward door, laden with presents as usual. Whenever I was in hospital, I would always receive an obscene amount of gifts. I was sitting with some other children when they came in and they took me back over to my bed immediately. Mum sat beside me and broke the news. Still giving nothing away, she told me very matter-of-fact that something was growing in my head that shouldn't be there. Putting on a brave face, she said the doctors were going to try and go inside my head to get it out.

I took the news rather better than she thought. I looked around the ward and saw the other children walking around with drips attached to their arms, some had shaven heads, signifying the chemotherapy treatment. It seemed everyone had something, a bandage or mark to show they belonged in the room. When mum told me I had a tumour I thought, 'Well, at least I'm the same as the rest of them.' I didn't feel left out.

Mum was determined to find more answers. She demanded another meeting with the consultant and neurosurgeon Mr Blaiklock. Mum pleaded, "Please look at the scan again. There must be something you can do." The surgeon replied that the tumour sat in an extremely difficult area of the brain to get to. And he explained the prognosis was nearly impossible to predict. Apparently I could drop tomorrow, next week or anytime. Mum asked again if my tumour was cancerous. He said it was at the lower end of the cancer spectrum but emphasised that anything growing on the brain of a young child that shouldn't be was harmful enough. In any event, he warned, non-malignant tumours could turn cancerous over night. Again he could give no guarantees and said it was unlikely he would be able to operate, but he recommended more scans and said if a way could be found, he would take it.

He explained the philosophy of neurosurgeons as regards tumours is to manage them, rather than eradicate them or remove them. Some, he said, simply cannot be removed because of the risk of damage to the patient. They have to be monitored closely. Brain tumours can go from being very benign to very malignant extremely quickly. Technically they are not brain tumours but growths of the grey matter's supporting cells, the bits that hold the brain together, rather than the thinking parts inside. The build-up of pressure in my brain had focused on the pineal gland, sitting in the middle that had caused swelling and prevented fluid from draining away as normal. What he had to work out was how best to manage my tumour.

All around the ward, the children, nurses and parents were taking part in a Halloween party. Mum despaired. Usually so strong after all we had been through together, she now scanned the room with tears in her eyes. Little boys, with tubes sticking out of them, were taking part in the games. Some were 'dooking' for apples. A nurse called over: "Come on and join in the fun." Mum was not in the mood for fun. Amazingly, the Nicols were there again. Vince was down on his hands and knees joining in the dooking games, trying to put a brave face on for his Caroline and the other children, even though his heart must have been breaking.

The Nicols had received slightly better news at that point. When surgeons detected Caroline's tumour, they were convinced it could be removed. As my friend was very poorly, doctors were anxious not to delay surgery and she was scheduled for an operation in the next few weeks. Mum would have given her right arm for some hope to cling to at that point, despite the risks surgery brings.

The next step for me, however, was another scan; this time a Magnetic Resonance Imaging Scan, or MRI. Formerly nuclear scans, Aberdeen had led the way in Scotland by being one of the first places to test drive the new technology. The MRI, which only shows soft tissue and is not distorted by bone like its CT counterpart, almost literally shed more light on the situation. Its scan showed the tumour bigger, this time three centimetres in diameter.

Over the next few weeks, mum pestered Mr Blaiklock and the other consultants to give me the same chance they appeared to be giving Caroline. It was not a case of like for like, mum just simply refused to believe nothing could be done to sort this. Several times though, his answer was no. He simply could not find a way into the brain.

Then, out of the blue, he said he had studied the scans again and now wanted me to take an angiogram, an x-ray of the blood vessels inside the brain. If the vessels were behaving accordingly he said, then he thought he had found a way into the tumour. Such surgery had great risks, he stressed. I could be blinded, paralysed, or worse. On the other hand, though, I might yet get to blow ten candles out on my birthday cake.

"You beauty," though mum. She was delighted. If he had said he would have to cut an ear off to get in, she would have said: "Go for it!"

The surgeon scheduled me for my third brain operation in as many years later that month. The plan was to remove my pineal gland and, with it, the tumour growing on my brain.

Chapter Eight
Going In

The Pineal gland is a small reddish-grey body sitting in the middle of the brain, right between the two hemispheres. This sausage-shaped organ grows large in children, before reducing to only about 8mm in diameter after puberty in adults. Although the gland performs several vital functions in animals, most importantly regulating their reproductive cycles and hibernation, its importance in humans is the subject of some debate. Reptiles and birds use the pineal gland as a "third eye", setting their body clocks by the light from the sun. Yet in humans, its chief role is in the production of melatonin, a hormone that may influence our sleep cycles. Dubbed by some physiologists as the "master hormone" because it helps keep all the others in check, there have been many arguments about its true worth to us. Some say melatonin helps combat diseases and it enjoys increasing popularity as a dietary supplement, while others claim it can have an even greater role by assisting in the fight against cancers, HIV and dementia. Despite this, very few clinical trials have been carried out into its effectiveness in this role.

In my case, fate had simply decided this misunderstood gland would be the perfect place to hide a tumour. As I said, each scan I'd had since they diagnosed my hydrocephalus gave doctors cause for concern. They were convinced something in my brain was causing the blockage and the pressure to build. They just could not see what. It had taken a combination of a CT scan and an MRI image to reveal finally what was behind my problems.

When Mr Blaiklock announced he believed there was a way in to get it, mum was thrilled. Although devastated at the grave danger I was in, she prayed surgery might give me the life the tumour had denied me since the age of five. Exploratory tests were done to establish there were no abnormalities in the vessels around the pineal gland. Once the results gave me the all-clear, the neurosurgeon was all set to begin. I was readmitted for surgery on 20th November 1990, less than a month since they had detected the tumour.

By now, we had a bit of a routine going. It was a tradition that before all my operations, mum enlisted the help of Rob's cousin Averil, who worked as a hairdresser. I hated having my hair cut at all but I accepted it was easier for the surgeons to operate and it did not seem as big a sacrifice to have a little hair trimmed once I was in hospital rather than see it hacked off in lumps. Averil would come into the ward and calmly snip off all my beautiful locks. However, just because I could see the sense in it, it did not mean I was happy with it.

The rest of the family, by this time, had grown used to me being in hospital and my brother and sisters also soon settled into a routine that kicked into place whenever I was in Aberdeen. Rob would take Michael, Dorothy and Averil to stay at a friend, Helen's, house, while mum would come through to Aberdeen with me. Rob would do his best to make the journey once he had cleared his workload but, more often than not, needed to be back in Dufftown after visits to see his clients. It was not an ideal situation but the family rallied round and soon these exceptional circumstances became the normality.

Brain operations, like the one performed on me, are extremely rare. Mr Blaiklock, my neurosurgeon, has only carried out a handful in his long and distinguished career. They are not taken lightly. The consultants once again outlined to mum and Rob the substantial risks with such a procedure. The outlook was bleak. I could be crippled and spend the rest of my life confined to a wheelchair. I could lose my sight or other senses or, worst of all, I could be left permanently brain damaged. With potential worst-case scenarios like those, it seems incredible these were the preferred options as opposed to complete inaction. Doing nothing could mean my young life cut short.

"I'll take any of that," mum reassured herself, "as long as she is alive."

Despite the risks, in the lead up to the surgery I told myself I was a dab hand at this. I tried to convince myself I knew what was in store for me and tried to bolster my confidence by thinking how I had taken previous operations in my stride. I did not fully understand what was going on of course. Instinctively you know the situation is pretty serious but I doubt I really knew precisely what was at stake. Mum, Rob and the staff at the hospital preferred not to dwell on the negative. It was always just explained to me that the operation was a simple case of a man going into my head to pluck out something that should not be there.

A piece of cake… happens every day.

Yet sometimes people can be too flippant about a situation and the more effort put into making me feel better started to have the opposite effect. I began to notice a nervous twinge, deep in my stomach.

Back then I was just a little slip of a girl, there was nothing to me. (But believe me I'm making up for it now!) Yet, mum had always marvelled at how well I seemed to deal with the adversity thrown at me on a regular basis. While other parents reported how their children screamed to the heavens when the time came to administer the anaesthetic, I surprised everyone by how calm I remained. However, the closer it got to the big day, the more nervous I became. I may not have been a brain surgeon, had the benefit of scans or the know-how to decipher them, but I knew my own body and intuitively sensed this was not going to be a walk in the park.

So, when it came to the day of the operation, I was very scared. Mum was terrified too and, although she was doing her best to hide it, I could detect her anxiety and that made me all the more nervous. I kept saying to mum, "Are you going to come with me to the theatre? Will you stay with me until they put me to sleep?" All the while, she said yes, of course she would. She assured me she would be with me all the time. In fact, and to her despair, the medics would not allow her to come with me.

Yet again I was making the journey from the children's hospital by ambulance to Ward Forty in the main infirmary. To a young child the corridors in the main hospital were huge and the smell of disinfectant made my eyes water. The ward was split into sections, segregated by sex. Here I was out of the relative comfort zone of the children's ward and into the real world. Sandwiched between women aged twenty to eighty. I suddenly felt seriously ill. All too soon it was time for the main event. Mum followed me to the theatre but had to watch as they wheeled me away for the anaesthetic. She stared after me, scarcely believing this was my third major operation. This was not the life she had imagined for me. When I had been gravely ill with hydrocephalus three years previously she prayed for an end to my suffering. This time, as the theatre doors swung shut, she feared it would be the last time she saw me alive.

The surgeon chose to perform the operation with me sitting up. He preferred this to me lying on my back because the blood would run down and away from vital organs. I am not one to spare the gory details so I can tell you he went in through the gap above the cerebellum at the back of the head, through a membrane, across the two hemispheres and into the pineal gland. Apparently, in surgery stakes, the inner sanctum of the brain is not the easiest place to get to, being virtually right in the centre of the skull.

Once inside my brain, one of the immediate things that struck the surgeon when he found the pineal gland was that it was bigger than it should be. Around the gland he could see dense arachnoid tissue, membranes containing the central nervous system and he saw the great vein of Galan, one of the major blood vessels that drain the skull, surrounded by smaller veins passing to the temporal lobes on either side. I suppose the biggest shock for my family was that he had found a brain at all!

After assessing the landscape, he could not see an obvious abnormality that could measure two to three centimetres – such as was shown in the scans. He looked again at the pineal region. The tumour must be inside the swollen gland. His options were limited. He decided to remove the gland entirely, taking care not to damage adjacent cerebral veins. Confident he had removed the lot, he patched me back up and waited to see what effects the invasive surgery would have on his patient.

For the duration of the five hour operation, mum had been pacing the corridors, pestering the nurses for answers, willing them to put her out of her misery. Thankfully, this time there was no agonising wait as before, and in no time mum received the news she had been waiting for. I was out of theatre and in

47

recovery. Mum rushed down to see me. She wanted to make sure hers would be the first face I saw when I woke up. She did not want me to see a stranger's faces when I opened my eyes. For her, it was such a relief when I slowly opened my eyes. I don't remember much about waking up from that operation but I do recall being able to see almost straight away, albeit blurry and fuzzed. I told mum I could see her and managed to squeeze out the hint of a smile. The next sensation I felt was a raindrop on my mouth. I licked my lips and was at first puzzled by the salty taste. It was not rain. It was a tear. Looking up, I saw mums eyes welling up even though she was smiling broadly.

Mr Blaiklock came up to mum. He explained to mum how he believed the tumour was in the pineal gland and that he was confident he had got the lot. Mum was relieved. Although her girl was still very sick and would require a lot of care and attention to fully recover, surely this meant the worrying was over. She was saved. Surely?

Chapter Nine
Life on the Ward

We came up from recovery that afternoon. The hospital chaplain came to see me and I recognised him too, which was a big moment for mum and Rob. It demonstrated the surgery had not damaged my memory cells. They checked me over like a newborn baby. Nurses started testing my reflexes, making sure my fingers worked. When they moved to try my legs, mum's heart was in her mouth. This was the one they warned us about – that I might never walk again. A moment later, everyone around my bed gasped with delight when the feeling returned to my toes immediately.

The doctors were very kind. In what had become a bit of a tradition, they patched up my teddy bear, Percy, to show he had been through exactly what I had.

Mum rang through to her friend Helen, who was looking after Michael, Dorothy and Averil. Helen had been sitting by the phone anxiously awaiting news of the operation. Michael, eight-years-older than me, and no doubt revelling in his role as the man of the house to his little sisters, was equally concerned for my wellbeing. He was old enough to realise the seriousness of the situation. The same couldn't be said for Dorothy. It was almost impossible for her to grasp the enormity of the situation, simply because by then it was a normal thing for me to be in hospital. Yet when the call came in, she, like the rest of the family, was hugely relieved and could not wait to come though; if only to muscle in on all the new toys I would be getting!

As I've mentioned, there was never a shortage of gifts; whether from family or well-wishers back in Dufftown. Of course, I wasn't complaining! They helped take my mind off the scar at the back of my head and my patchwork hairdo, which by now made me look like a skunk that had picked a fight with a lawnmower. I sported a nice shaven strip down the middle of my head.

The presents were not the only reason I looked forward to visitors. I always loved seeing the rest of the family. Averil and Dorothy would treat the place like one big playroom and saw the hospital as an adventure playground. Grandpa and nana would come over from Skye with my uncle and his family, and Archie would make it over if work allowed.

My sisters thought it was exciting when Rob gave them money and allowed them to go to the hospital shop to buy snacks and sweets. Michael and Dorothy resumed playing in the wheelchairs, racing each other up and down the large corridors. The days following the operation were tiring. I was in a wheelchair at first and the reality was that I had a long road ahead of me back to full health.

I needed a lot of physiotherapy. Although the early indications were that the operation was a success and I had the use of my limbs, nurses had to basically teach me how to walk again. My joints were stiff and my legs and feet needed work. It was a slow process. The paediatrician warned us before the operation that it could leave lasting damage because it was serious brain surgery, so we had to play a patient, waiting game to see what effects the surgery would have on me. I could see but my sight was poorly and my speech slurred after the operation. In many ways, it was like I had suffered a stroke. My head slumped to one side after the operation because they had removed part of the bone supporting the back of my skull. Mum had to teach me to hold my head upright. She propped it up with a toilet roll, a trick she had learned while working in an old people's home.

It was an immensely tiring time for mum and Liz Nicol, who at the same time was awaiting news on Caroline's prognosis. Both mums were flattened and exhausted after the strain of the past few months. Not only were they required to play the supporting role for their daughters, keeping our spirits up and trying to remain positive, they also had to keep their fears hidden from us, while maintaining their strength for visitors and the rest of the families.

One night when they were both in the parents' sitting room after a particularly exhausting day, Liz said to mum, "Vince has a present for us." It was two miniature bottles of brandy and two bottles of ginger ale. With all they had been through a stiff drink was the least they deserved. In addition, after days of stomaching canteen food and water, the sight of the liquor – forbidden inside the hospital – was manna from heaven to mum. However, as they were about to find out, getting to taste it was another matter entirely.

The two women spent ages frantically trying to open the bottles because Vince had neglected to bring an opener. They scoured the room, searching for a suitable surface to lever the tops off. Vainly they tried the side of the table, possibly even marking it in the process. Surely these bottles were welded shut? Mum tried her teeth, and had a go on the windowsill but still the bottle tops would not budge. At that point, a ward sister entered the room. Both mums, thinking the staff nurse had rumbled them, instinctively sat down abruptly like naughty schoolchildren, their faces crimson with embarrassment. Mum panicked and hid the bottles in the only place she could think of – up her denim skirt. Terrified they were heading for fifty lashes, mum was scared to move and prayed the sister did not ask them to accompany her back down to the ward. She knew, as soon as she stood up, the bottles would tumble from their hiding place and smash on the floor. Frozen with fear, they waited, holding their breath until the sister finally left the room. Mum, heaving a sigh of relief, rescued the bottles and eventually managed to open them on the coffee machine. The two women, thrown together by such terrible circumstances, roared with laughter. Despite the ordeal they were going through, the moment of light relief was not lost on them and they drank in the moment just as heartily as they supped the sweet liquor. The golden brandy was like nature's purest nectar as it warmed their souls.

This was just momentary respite. For the most part, life in the hospital was unbearable for Liz and mum. Following the diagnosis, they found the most frustrating thing was getting to see a specialist to give them some nugget of news about our condition or perhaps a glimmer of hope. As the consultants carried out their rounds in the ward, parents would sit anxiously, not knowing if they would receive good news or any news at all. Sometimes, despite the fact the experts knew how tortuous each family's situation was, they would walk on by without so much as a cursory glance in your direction. If they did not have an update for you they were not interested, it seemed to be mean.

Soon mum was petrified to leave the ward, even to go to the canteen, in case she missed the specialist passing with a vital piece of information. She and Liz would take it in turns to sound the alarm that a doctor was doing the rounds.

Despite these imperfections, much was done on Ward Four to help the children and their families function as normally as possible on a day-to-day basis. For patients like me, we had a classroom set up in the children's ward to compensate for the days we were missing at school. Every morning staff called the children, including Caroline and me, for lessons. Nurses telephoned each patient's school to find the level they were at so they could tailor the classes accordingly. It was not ideal and I think some of the teaching methods dismayed my parents but the staff meant well. Their biggest problem was motivating the children. Trying to persuade a young boy or girl to go to school is a difficult task at the best of times but try doing it to a room full of sick kids with a dozen distractions and beds to seek refuge in.

The simple truth was, I could not be bothered with this makeshift classroom; especially not when there were so many toys around the place. I would always find an excuse for not going and coincidently always managed to time my toilet breaks perfectly with the start of the lessons. Then I would be off to check if the postman had been through the ward delivering even more cards and gifts – see what I mean about the distractions?

Caroline and I became thick as thieves. Often, when the teacher called us, we would lie flat on our backs in bed in the hope they would think us too sleepy to attend.

The weeks we spent in hospital before and after the operation were hard going. In a bid to relieve the boredom, mum would push me out of the children's hospital to get some fresh air. Sometimes we would go to the canteen for food but other times we would simply go for a walk to look at the gardens.

The canteen supplied welcome nourishment but we both quickly tired of the same standard issue sandwiches. I despaired at the hospital meals in general. They were always stone cold by the time they reached me and it seemed more like prison gruel than grub to help sick people get back on their feet. Mum was grateful for any food smuggled in from the outside and friends and family often came to the rescue. They would drive Mum to a local sandwich shop whose fare was a far preferable alternative; and like the alcohol she had shared with Liz in the parents' room; it was a slice of heaven.

When you are living 24/7 in a hospital ward, simple chores can become arduous tasks. Shortly after the operations, mum realised the pyjamas she had brought for me were unsuitable because they were all round-necked. As I could not yet pull clothes over my head because of the scar, she was keen to get me buttoned nightwear instead. One day she nipped out to complete what she thought would be a simple errand. Yet despite trawling through store after store, she could not find the right style. Care Bears were all the rage in those days and soon the sight of the cuddly creatures on t-shirt pyjamas almost drove her mental. Eventually it was nana that came up trumps in Skye.

Gradually mum started to go stir-crazy in the parents' room. If her pal Liz was not around, mum thought it a very depressing place and found it increasingly difficult to stay over on her own. With Rob having to be back in Dufftown to work, mum decided it was better to go home and spend time with her other children, who had sadly grown used to life at home without mum or their sister. Even if it meant leaving Aberdeen to drive the 52 miles back to Dufftown at ten o'clock returning at 8am the following morning, she thought it better for her sanity than staying on her own overnight in Aberdeen.

I didn't mind. I was quite happy in the ward. I felt safe. I had a team of nurses standing by in case anything went wrong and it was nice having people at your disposal. I felt important.

As November turned into December, so the nurses started decorating the ward in tinsel and card; it was the build-up to Christmas. On days when I was too ill to get out of bed, they would bring things over to me to play with. There was a video library on the ward to keep us kids occupied and we could watch shaky re-runs of Disney classics and other children's favourites.

Lying in hospital knowing the family were decorating the tree back home and, outside, people were preparing to celebrate with their loved ones, was hard. It was a sad ward but the nurses did all they could to try to cheer the place up. The nurses held a party for the children in the ward. Many, like me, were too sick to join in the fun but the minister came over to my bed with a present from Santa and that put a smile on my face.

Wherever possible, the consultants tried to let as many kids home for Christmas. I was lucky. Although I was still quite poorly and needed more physiotherapy to bring me back to full fitness, Mr Blaiklock said I was able to go home for the festivities. I would also be home in time for my birthday. Mum was ecstatic. She would have all the children for Christmas, including Robina from Skye. I was thrilled as well. After what seemed like an eternity, it was amazing I would be able to spend Christmas at home with the others.

Naturally everyone else was equally delighted and it seemed I came home to a hero's welcome. Everyone in the town was so kind; the news of the operation caused quite a stir in Dufftown and people were happy it had all gone well. In fact, my sisters were astonished at the mountain of presents, which piled up in the house. It helped that my return from hospital coincided with my ninth birthday but I have always been touched by the interest and concern shown by relative strangers to my situation and the good wishes of neighbours and friends was never taken for granted.

For my birthday, we held a big party, inviting my friends from school, neighbours and all the family. Mum's friend, Helen, supplied the cake. It was a day I never dreamed I would be able to enjoy just two weeks before.

Chapter Ten
The Best of Times, the Worst of Times

The support network for children suffering from cancers and other horrific illnesses is astonishing in this country. Not only are we blessed with some of the sharpest medical minds working in our health service but, behind the scenes, charity workers toil tirelessly to mop up the pieces after operations or courses of treatment.

We were astounded by the support from a number of organisations whose job it is to help put families back on their feet when they have to come to terms with such devastating circumstances. Malcolm Sargent, the charity founded in 1967 to help the families of children with cancers, offered us a free holiday shortly after the operation to help recuperate from the trauma we had shared. Even though, strictly, I should not have qualified because my tumour was not really cancerous as such, the charity was only too willing to help. As it was, mum politely declined, feeling we were in the privileged position of being able to afford our own holidays. She hoped someone else would benefit from the generous offer.

In addition, we always received great support from Cancer Research. Robert Young, chairman of the charity in Scotland, liked to set up special events for sufferers of cancer and people affected by tumours. Grateful for the huge donations which had been winging his way from Dufftown – far outperforming the rest of the UK for donations per head of population – he arranged it for me to visit Ibrox stadium in Glasgow, the home of Rangers football club.

Like many ten-year-old girls, I was more interested in pop music than football and, ordinarily, would not have thought much of an offer for a stadium tour. However, despite showing no interest in football, I knew Rangers were different. A trip to Glasgow might mean I would get the chance to meet their star striker, Ally McCoist. He was dishy! Shortly after the tumour operation, I travelled to the big city with mum, Rob, Dorothy and Averil. The Rangers' staff gave us the star treatment when we arrived and went out of their way to make us feel very special. After a tour of the stadium, we were introduced to two of the players, Mo Johnston (who had caused fury amongst the fans of their greatest rivals Celtic by switching allegiances and signing for Rangers) and Ally McCoist, or Super Ally, as he was nicknamed. I was thrilled. He was so charming and took such an interest in my condition, wanting to hear all about it. Averil, being a big Celtic fan, was more interested in Mo, who had enjoyed a glittering career with the Boys before controversially becoming the first high-profile Catholic player to sign for Rangers. Yet that suited me fine. It meant I had Ally all to myself.

Mr Young was very kind to lots of children affected by cancer and I was not the only one to benefit from the charity's work. He arranged for Caroline Nicol to see Australian heartthrob and chart-topper Jason Donovan when she was quite poorly. Sadly, because she was confined to a wheelchair, she was not able to make it backstage to meet her hero, which was what had initially been arranged. Even though she was not able to meet the former Neighbours star, she still thoroughly enjoyed the concert in London.

I cannot underestimate the impact trips like those can have on a child stricken with cancer or a tumour. Once diagnosed with such a terrible condition, you are left with your own thoughts, the majority of them morbid. When you are young the last thing you contemplate is how long you will live for or, if you do, it is only to daydream about how many children and grandchildren you will have before you peacefully pass away in your cottage with a picket fence, your heart warmed by the memories of your happy life.

Suddenly you are given a dose of reality, as if someone has just started a stopwatch counting down the moments until you shuffle off this mortal coil. You feel nothing positive will come of your condition and never again will you feel the sensation of looking forward to something exciting. That is when the little trips and visits make all the difference. They take children out of themselves and, for a few short hours or days, make them forget what it was that brought them there. For a brief moment, we feel like *we* are the celebrities and strangely blessed for being in a position other children might give their back teeth for. Believe me, it is best to enjoy these moments while we can because we never know what's waiting for us round the corner.

I can only speak from experience of course… because that is exactly how it happened for me. After the tumour was removed, tests were done to examine exactly what it was inside my head that had been causing all the trouble. Although there was great debate about exactly what had caused the initial hydrocephalus, it was accepted that a tumour, in the pineal gland had enlarged the organ, causing the blockage and the subsequent build-up of pressure. Yet, while it was a relief to have me home, mum and Rob knew I was not out of the woods. It would be a while before I was strong enough or able to do things normal children my age took for granted.

After a few weeks of rest and recuperation at home, mum decided it was time for me to return to school. I had missed so much and, although I had been going to the classes occasionally in hospital, it did not compensate for being in class and working at the pace of the other kids.

Once again, when I returned to school, I was something of a novelty. My hair was shaven and I sported a nice scar on the back of my head. The country was still in the grip of winter and the highlands were a chilly place to be. Sometimes, shortly after I first went back, it was so bitterly cold at lunch and playtimes that I was not allowed outside. My classmates were asked to take it in turns to sit with me while the rest played outside. Boy, I must have been popular.

It was clear, though, what effect the lay-off had on my schooling. At the age I was, children advance in educational ability in leaps and bounds; after missing so many classes, it was not going to be easy to pick up where I left off. I quickly realised the tumour had not just had a physical impact on my life. Even though it was gone, the implications of its presence would be felt for some time yet. Not only had I missed school in the weeks following the operation but now the consequences of slipping away for hospital visits or taking the odd day here and there because of excruciating headaches were beginning to take their toll. In addition, the simple act of staying alert for a full school day after weeks of resting in a hospital bed seemed beyond me. The tiredness that had affected me so badly before the operation was still with me and, in many ways, it was difficult to see how removing the tumour had changed my life for the better.

Worryingly, the wearier I became, the more blurred my vision. After being told my deteriorating eyesight was a symptom of the lesion on my brain before surgery the previous November, I wondered what could be causing it now. Next, the headaches that had plagued my life for so many years, started to return, heavier and denser than before.

I began to feel like I was in a time warp. Surely I should be getting better? Hadn't the doctors been inside my head to fix it? It might have been simple, childlike logic from a nine-year-old, but for mum it made sense. Why was there no improvement?

She consulted with our local GP, Dr Heneghan who referred me once again to the specialists in Aberdeen. They were reluctant to schedule me for further scans because of the risks the exposure to radiation in the x-ray machines carried. They did not want to deviate from the course of treatment mapped out for me and initially refused to budge from the date set for my routine scan in June. They claimed there were few neurological signs to suggest anything more sinister than the hydrocephalus already diagnosed. Plus, they argued, hadn't a surgeon been inside my brain? If there had been a second tumour, they would have spotted it.

I think, reading between the lines, what they were saying was medical-speak for 'You're at it'.

However, mum persisted and, on 12th March 1991, I underwent the sixth scan on my brain. Here we were again, suffering the excruciating wait for scan results. With this one especially, they seemed to take an age to tell us. Maybe it was because the consultants had difficulty interpreting the information. Maybe there was some argument about what the scans showed. We did not know. All we knew was that the longer it went on without knowing the more desperate we became.

Then it was time. Dr Heneghan was the first to let us know. As our local doctor, he was more in tune with the anxieties of his patients and wanted us to know as soon as possible. He told us the scan had shown up an abnormality on the brain. He was not privy to the conclusions of the experts in Aberdeen, who duly summoned us back to the Granite City for the results.

It was far worse than failing an exam. They had found a shadow.

The scan picked up a small halo on the upper midbrain, the abnormality Dr Heneghan spoke of. Mr Blaiklock suspected it might be another tumour but there were doubts. One thing he did know though was that, if indeed, it proved to be a second lesion, this time there would be no operation. The chances of a successful procedure removing a tumour without damaging the sensitive veins and grey matter around it were virtually impossible.

It was too much to take. There were so many questions and the consultants did their best to give us answers. Yet they couldn't tell us why this was happening. Mum was beside herself. This was too much. To have gone through what we had been through as a family; the health problems, the water on the brain, having the shunt fitted, then the tumour followed by elation after surgeons removed it. Now this…

I sat motionless. Mr Blaiklock was the surgeon entrusted with the difficult job of explaining the situation. It must have been incredibly harrowing for him since he had been the one to go inside my head and take out what he thought was the entire growth. He tried to explain that there was a good chance what was showing up on the scan was not in fact a tumour. That was not good enough for mum. She demanded a second opinion. Reacting as any mother would, she felt guesswork and probabilities did not come into it where her daughter's health was concerned.

We left Aberdeen that day lower than we had ever been. It seemed everything was for nothing. The next few weeks were torture. Until the diagnosis was confirmed, we were in limbo. We did not know whether the growth was cancerous, how aggressive it might be and what my prognosis was.

The scan was sent to Dr Derek Kingsley, consultant neuro-radiologist at the Hospital for Sick Children at Great Ormond Street in London. His response a month later confirmed what we already feared. He said the only diagnosis to be entertained was that it was a tumour. His assessment concurred with Mr Blaiklock's opinion.

It seemed I had a second tumour, one that only decided to show itself after the operation to excise the first. Mr Blaiklock's view was that it was an astrocytoma. No, I had no idea what that meant at the time either. I'm an expert on it now.

An astrocytoma is a tumour that attacks the astrocytes – cells that are almost like the worker bees inside the head, structurally supporting the brain whilst also providing vital nutrients to the cells of the central nervous system. It is the most common form of brain tumour in children and it has a tendency to come back – something they never told me six months ago. Its position was on the upper midbrain, a part that leads to the stem and one of the most dangerous places in the head to operate. There was no chance of removing it.

I could not believe it. I had jumped from the proverbial frying pan right into the hottest furnace imaginable. Suddenly my life hung in the balance once again but, unlike last time, there would be no miracle cure.

The consultants tried to put a positive spin on the situation. It was a low-grade astrocytoma. That meant on a scale of one to four, I was a one and therefore stood the greatest chance of surviving past a year. That was the best-case scenario. The worst? I would still be lucky to see my tenth birthday, by now only seven months away.

To say the news was a kick in the teeth for mum and Rob was the understatement of the year. They were gutted. All the times they had prayed for an end to this nightmare were now, it seemed, for nothing. For mum, it was almost too much. The joy she had felt, just a few weeks earlier at getting me home for Christmas seemed like a lifetime ago. Trauma like this was supposed to be exclusive to other people's kids, not hers. This was like a script from a tragic B-movie – just when the heroine thinks she's come out on top the rug is pulled from under her and she is right back where she started.

In the time from the initial concern over the scan to the confirmation, I had feared the worst, but had always held a little back. Secretly I was convinced everything would be okay. This was just a scare, I told myself; a little panic before I get the all clear. It was unthinkable that, for the rest of my days on this Earth, I would have to live with a tumour inside my head.

I remember locking myself in a toilet for an hour after we got the confirmation; sobbing, inconsolable. I demanded answers from a higher authority. Why me? Why was I the one to be put through such misery? What had I done to deserve this? I convinced myself I must have done some serious damage in a past life. This was not normal – to be put through so much at such a young age and over such a brief period of time. I hadn't even had the chance to enjoy life since the operation. It was almost as though the tumour was waiting for the first opportunity once I was back on my feet and, then wham! Handle that…

I honestly believed the Gods were dealing me such terrible hands out of spite.

We had regular meetings with our doctor and the consultants. Their advice might have been practical but, for a nine-year-old girl it was not what I wanted to hear. They repeated that they could not operate this time. I challenged them. That's what they'd said last year and then they had found a way in. "Go in and do it again." I said. "Take it out."

Poor Mr Blaiklock; a tremendous surgeon who had probably saved my life, he must have been taken aback by my directness.

But, hey, this was my brain, my tumour and my life they were talking about.

Still their answer was the same. This was different. It would be too difficult to go in through the thickest part of the skull at the back of the head and then, once inside, they had no way of predicting what they would find. They told me all they could do was monitor the tumour's growth. I was entering a watch and wait phase. I would have to come to terms with the idea I had something growing inside my brain that would be with me forever. Up until that point, this was something I had never considered. When surgeons identified the original growth in November I had no time to come to terms with what it meant before they were scheduling me for surgery to have it removed. Now I would have to grow up all of a sudden.

The thought of living with a foreign entity, growing in my head that could one day kill me filled me with horror. The more

I thought about it, the more panicked I became. And in December, just four days before my tenth birthday – the landmark day surgeons feared I'd never see – I received news that would send my life spiralling out of control; news that terrified me so much, it was as if someone had just started the clock on the countdown to my death.

Chapter Eleven
Caroline Nicol

Caroline was the first child born to Vince and Liz Nicol. The first granddaughter in their extended family, she was doted on from the moment she arrived on 23rd June 1982, just six months after I entered the world. Popular Elgin couple Liz and Vince, a maths teacher at Lossiemouth High School and a bar manager, had their work cut out dealing with the sparkling new edition to the family but, with both sets of grandparents close by there was always an extra pair of hands to help out.

To say Caroline was much like any other girl would be doing her a huge disservice. She was beautiful; with golden locks I could only dream of and a bubbly personality to light up any room she graced. Caroline doted on her youngster sister, Kirsty, born two years after her. Ironically it was Kirsty who was given little chance of survival after a traumatic birth.

During her second pregnancy, midwives stunned Liz by discovering she was expecting quads. Heartbreakingly, one failed to survive and Liz suffered a miscarriage just weeks into the pregnancy. As it was, none of the babies would last full-term because Liz started having contractions at only 28 weeks. She was taken through to Aberdeen Royal Infirmary where surgeons advised an emergency caesarean section. Miraculously Liz gave birth to all three babies, although their condition was perilous. Two weighed not much more than a kilogram, while Kirsty, the last to be delivered, touched just 910 grams on the scales. The eldest, Christopher, and the second born, Lorna, battled bravely for life after their birth on 30th August 1983. Tragically Christopher died two days later, and Lorna followed shortly after on 5th September.

However Kirsty, so fragile she resembled a tiny rag doll, had the heart of a lion and, to the amazement of doctors at the hospital, pulled through. Moreover, as I write this, she recently celebrated her 22nd birthday.

The Nicols would have been forgiven for believing the gods had finished their sport with the family after that harrowing ordeal, but it was not to be. Caroline was to call upon the same courage shown by her infant sister when fate decided to take a hand in her life.

The youngster was just eight, with her whole life ahead of her, when Liz got the call at school from her teacher to say something was wrong with her eldest daughter. By the time her frantic mum got to the local primary, Caroline was ashen white. She was hurried over to her GP who dismissed the symptoms as an extreme reaction to a particularly nasty virus doing the rounds. Her head was bursting. At one stage the pain was so unbearable she tried to bang her skull against the sofa in a desperate bid to end her misery. Doctor after doctor visited the house. One prescribed penicillin. She couldn't eat or drink anything. Anything she did consume was rejected quickly afterwards.

Caroline battled on though and, seemingly feeling a little better, started school again. Cruelly though, for all her family's praying that she'd turned the corner, it was a false dawn. Before too long her teachers rang Liz again. She'd taken another turn for the worse. Again medics were summoned to the house but they were no closer to establishing exactly what was paralysing this previously healthy eight-year-old girl.

Then, while Liz was bathing her one night, Caroline had a seizure. Vince rushed home. They were told to take her through to Aberdeen as soon as possible. Within minutes of her arriving, specialists spotted the pressure building behind her eyes and, within half an hour of being admitted, Caroline was being whisked for surgery to insert her shunt.

Like me, she had hydrocephalus and, like the early stages of my condition, doctors struggled to trace the source of the blockage. They did not know it then but a tumour was stopping the flow of fluid from the brain.

After the operation, the change was remarkable. Caroline's colour improved almost immediately. As most little girls would be, she was devastated her long blonde hair had gone – she was especially proud of her locks. But she was sitting up in bed and looked a lot better. In the weeks that followed she even recovered enough to go back to school at Elgin East End primary, where her teachers worked overtime to make her feel less self-conscious. They encouraged her to take off her hat, to talk about her operation and show the other kids her scar.

Just when Liz and Vince dared to think their angel was out of the woods, Caroline started to complain of the same symptoms again. Her parents believed her shunt must have blocked. One of the local GPs arrived and she was taken back through to Aberdeen Royal Infirmary. Surgeons revised the valve in her brain but she was sent for a routine post-operative MRI scan.

This time it picked up the tumour. Liz and Vince were taken into a little room and, while her maternal instinct was probably enough for her to know something terrible was happening, Liz knew the minute staff offered them tea and biscuits it could only be bad news.

They said there was a distortion in the tube. They had the MRI scan and said it had picked up an astrocytoma – a starfish-like tumour with legs stretching to several parts of the brain. The growth was on the brain stem. The prognosis was not good. At best, she might see three more Christmases. A glimmer of hope was that they believed they could operate. There was no time to lose and surgeons scheduled Caroline for surgery almost immediately. Staff emphasised the risks attached to such an operation. She might go blind or lose the use of her limbs. Yet without surgery the prognosis was grim. Caroline was prepared for the operation while Liz and Vince prayed for a miracle.

It was only when surgeons were inside Caroline's head they realised the futility of the operation. The tumour was too large. The chances of removing it without causing irreparable damage to vital organs were practically non-existent. She would almost certainly be paralysed or left with severe brain damage.

With heavy hearts, the operation was halted.

As if the Nicols had not suffered enough on this rollercoaster of emotions and false hope, they were offered one last throw of the dice. A neurosurgeon, based seventy miles away in Dundee, was using a new method relying on the latest computer technology. They had no choice but to pin all their hopes on further surgery. The brave youngster, still just nine years old, travelled to the City of Discovery for the operation and again she went under the surgeon's knife. But again, this time after only half an hour, he decided not to proceed further.

To their credit, the experts in Aberdeen, despite the odds stacked against them, looked for possible solutions all the time. First it was decided to try radiotherapy. Liz, determined her daughter would feel the benefit of as much time at home as possible, decided to take her to and from Aberdeen for treatment rather than have Caroline spend weeks on end in a strange hospital.

Liz and Vince had already discussed with the specialists whether it was a good idea to tell Caroline and had settled on the tactic that it was better not to explain too much about what was exactly happening to her. However, Caroline was a smart girl and, in herself, she knew she was seriously unwell. In one heart-wrenching moment Caroline, rather matter-of-fact, asked her mum not to spend money on new clothes for her – she knew they would not be needed.

Whenever she was required to stay over at the Craig Unit, in the children's hospital, with Liz sleeping in the family quarters, it was Vince who, like Rob for me, was left with the horrendous return trips between Elgin and Aberdeen. The strain took its toll in near-fatal consequences as late one night, and exhausted; he fell asleep at the wheel. The car mounted a grass verge and crossed the other side of the carriageway before veering back into the lane he was travelling in. Only the deserted roads saved him from joining his daughter in the hospital.

As it was, the radiotherapy made little progress. The consultants said chemotherapy was an option but they feared the impact it would have on the tumour was negligible and was not worth the sickness it would cause her. The next step was to put a tap in her shunt to relieve the pressure and at least give her some respite from the crippling headaches and impaired sight. Sadly, like everything else tried on Caroline, it fell short of what was needed. Her health deteriorated rapidly. She started to feel weak down her left side.

The inevitable came when the consultant paediatric neurosurgeon admitted there was nothing more the health service could do for Caroline. She told her parents to take her home. If they were lucky, they would probably have just two weeks left as a family.

It could not have been more heartbreaking for Liz and Vince, being forced to watch their beloved daughter slip away, powerless to do anything to stop it.

As Caroline became weaker and weaker, everyday tasks were beyond her. A simple game of Happy Families with friends proved too much when she was unable to focus on the cards. Although now confined to a wheelchair, Caroline continued to battle on and enjoyed accompanying Liz to the shops to meet people. Soon, however, even those trips started to have a detrimental effect when her eyes failed her and she found it impossible to identify once familiar voices. Riddled with pain, she was prescribed morphine to make her last days as bearable as possible but having to administer it pushed Liz's sanity to the limit. Fortunately a neighbour, Ann Glover, was a district nurse who kindly offered her services day and night to handle the tasks that would have tested any parent's resolve.

It was nearly impossible for the family and they prayed for anything other than to watch their child suffer in such a manner. Yet, through even this, Caroline remained as cheerful as was humanly possible.

But even she could not delay the inevitable. When the call came, Vince was at work. By the time he arrived home, Caroline was lying on the sofa; she was on her last legs. When the moment came, Liz and Vince could only watch as the colour drained from their daughter's face. Showing remarkable courage, they took comfort from the fact Caroline was spared the pain that had plagued her last days when she finally slipped away.

Vince served in the Royal Air Force and was stationed in Northern Ireland at the height of the Troubles for two years. He has seen a lot in this world. But the thought of seeing his girl fighting for her life still breaks his heart 15 years on.

Caroline Nicol died just three weeks from the day she came home from hospital, on 9th October 1991; nearly a year from the day we were both diagnosed with brain tumours. She was nine years old.

Her death had a profound effect on me. I did not understand it. She was the same age as me, had the same name, and the same tumour. I kept asking myself, 'Why was it not me?'

Mum visited the Nicols the day before Caroline passed away and attended the funeral; a heart-wrenching day for her distraught family. She and Liz had grown so close during their time spent together in the hospital. The Nicols came to visit me when I was discharged and the families remained close.

Her death terrified me. It meant this thing was real. This was not a game. All I kept thinking was, 'How long do I have?'

This fear was to shape my life for the next two years and my paranoia would push our family to breaking point.

Chapter Twelve
A Day They Said I Would Never See

Two months after Caroline's death, I was blowing out ten candles on my birthday cake. It was a bittersweet moment. The joy everyone in the family felt that I had reached this symbolic day was tempered with the sadness that, just twenty miles up the road, another family were still mourning the passing of their little girl.

I was not prepared for the response of local people to my predicament. News of the tumour had spread around the town and locals had reacted in the most positive ways. Everyone was concerned for my wellbeing and determined to mark the birthday I thought I might never see.

Mum desperately wanted to hold a party but she was still reeling from everything that had happened in the previous months and was in no fit state to organise it. That job fell to our good friend, Hazel Massie, who ran the local whisky shop with her husband. Hazel was a tower of strength to mum during the dark days in hospital and volunteered to help with the party. It was to be held in the town's Memorial Hall, the setting for the family's now annual Cancer Research fund-raisers. Since mum and Rob had got involved with the charity two years previously, she had come up with the idea of holding a two-day event each year to raise as much money as possible for people whose lives had been touched by the terrible disease. It was a real family affair as mum was secretary of the local branch, with Rob chairman.

The events had been an amazing success. Each year, over two nights, mum and her friends would organise a cabaret of entertainment. They were always themed. One year it would be musicals, the next wartime songs, another time a take-off of Top of the Pops or Jukebox Jury. The previous year, in 1990, it had been based on the World Cup, taking place that summer in Italy. Scotland had qualified for the finals and the event was timed to coincide with the nation's opening game against South American minnows Costa Rica. Of course, the festivities were expected to follow on from a famous win that would set us up to qualify from the group stages for the first time in our history. Sadly, yet predictably and not for the first time, our heroes let us down and crashed 1-0 to the Latin nobodies. Still, it failed to dampen our spirits and, if anything, the adverse result generated more takings at the bar as patriotic locals drowned their sorrows!

Whenever possible, the whole family mucked in and it was great fun helping to make the costumes and rehearse the musical numbers. Lots of people in the town joined in and the events caught everyone's imagination.

Thousands of pounds were raised for charity through the celebrations and, one year the branch won the prestigious Nuffield Award for being the top fundraisers for the year. The family were celebrating the following year too, when the Skye branch, where my uncle was an office bearer, topped the pile for Britain.

The annual event had been running since 1989, before I became ill, and it was already a fixture on the local calendar. I do not know if that had a bearing on my situation, but once again neighbours and friends rallied round to put on a wonderful party for yours truly. Hazel, who was a veteran of the cancer events, organised the catering for my grateful mum, who I think would have found the whole event much too emotional. It was a fantastic day – one I'll cherish forever – with all my family and friends around me. A huge banner adorned the wall proclaiming "Happy 10th Birthday Caroline".

As a wonderful surprise, nana and grandpa arrived from Skye but the biggest gasp of the day was reserved for Santa, who made a guest appearance, dispensing presents for all the children.

As I said, the closeness of Caroline's death meant she was never far from my thoughts but at least I was able to put aside my worries for a short time and enjoy the moment.

The happiness that united the family was short-lived, however, as, away from the celebrations and festivities, we were going through our living nightmare – and I was responsible for it all.

The seeds of insecurity had been planted in my mind before Caroline's death but, since she passed away, I became obsessed with my own mortality. Back in the house in Scorrybreck, with only my parents and brother and sisters for company, I started to feel strangely cut off from my medical support unit. In hospital I had felt safe, secure in the knowledge that if my condition deteriorated overnight, nurses and doctors were on hand to come to my assistance. Now, at home, there was no such back - up. If anything were to happen, it was a long way back to Aberdeen.

The symptoms had come on much like they had five years ago. The headaches, with which I should now have been accustomed, returned with a vengeance; especially in the morning. They paralysed me with pain, shooting sharp shocks round the front of my skull. Then the pain started to spread to other parts of my body. I suffered a sore back, sore eyes and the tiredness that had crippled me before my operation returned once more.

The consultants were baffled. Neurologically I was fine. I was putting on weight following the operation, my reflexes were good and I passed all the tests used to identify brain disorders. Emotionally though I was a wreck. I was sharing a room with Averil at the time my sleeping problems began. Almost without warning, I became scared to go to sleep. I was worried I would never wake up. What had happened to Caroline had really shaken me up.

If I did manage to get to sleep I would wake up in a panic, drenched in sweat and frightened; unsure where I was and what had happened since I had last been awake.

Quickly, I developed severe, obsessive-compulsive habits. Subconsciously I transferred my health fears into general paranoia about our safety. Sometimes I would lie in bed and be convinced that the house was not locked properly. I would shout through to dad, mostly after he had gone to bed, "Have you locked the front door?" If he did not respond, I obsessed about doing the job myself. Getting up after the last person had gone to bed. I had to make sure the doors were shut, again and again and again. Even though I could hear the handle click in the lock, I continued pushing on the door until my arm bruised.

If I did drop off to sleep, eventually I would wake up to find I had wet the bed.

Soon, I was driving everyone in the house mad, as I called out in the darkness late at night, "Dad, are the lights out? Is the cooker switched off?" The silence would be disrupted further by a chorus of: "Caroline, shut up! Caroline. Go to sleep!"

Every night, almost without fail, the others would be kept awake as I shouted through the house about my various insecurities. Despite my sleeping problems, I continued to be sent to bed early, at 8 o'clock on the dot and be forced to lie awake. Lying awake only gave me more time to develop more behavioural problems.

I am sure that when Mr Blaiklock removed the pineal gland from my head, he also took my thermometer because I became convinced I was shivering with cold when the house was roasting hot. When mum came through to check on me, she was shocked to see me buried under a mountain of sheets, blankets and duvets, saturated with sweat. And when mum peeled back the covers, she was bewildered to find the Monopoly board, the Sellotape dispenser and an array of other household items buried under the sheets with me. Don't ask me to explain, but I was convinced they would be feeling the cold too.

Other times I drove mum mad by getting up and emptying the linen cupboard to insulate the bed. On top of the covers would go freshly pressed sheets, towels, Rob's shirts for work, and anything else I could lay my hands on; piling them up on top of the duvet, sometimes as high as about 4ft off the bed, with me sitting perched at the top.

As you can imagine, my behavioural quirks were not endearing me to the rest of the household. Mum took me out of the room I shared with Averil and, for a while, I slept with her and Rob on a chair bed in their room. That did not work either. Every night, just as dad finished working in his office and crept into bed, I would pipe up; "Dad, can you make sure everything is off? Dad, are the hamsters warm enough?" I would lie there in the dark asking dad if he had checked everything was off. He would have to get up and check it all for me.

During the day I would not be much better. I felt very clingy to mum and became terrified at the thought of her leaving the house. I don't know if it was a reaction to the reality that I was now having to share her with the other children, whereas in the hospital I enjoyed her exclusive attention. Whatever the reason, I used to grab mum round the neck whenever she tried to leave the house, sometimes gripping on so tightly I would leave scratch marks on her neck. If she still made to leave after that I would scream the house down until she relented.

Other times, I would hide her bras and knickers so she could not leave the house without turning everything upside down to find them. Or, I would squirrel away the car keys for the same reason. It drove mum to distraction.

It sounds ridiculous behaviour now but, at the time, it all seemed very rational. It did not help that my sisters relentlessly bullied me.

Any sympathy I garnered during my stays in hospital had evaporated with my nightly antics. In addition, I would infuriate them further when I was excused from running errands because of my health problems. Children see things in black and white and when they see a girl fit enough to go to school but deemed too fragile to nip to the shop for some potatoes, they feel a deep-seated injustice.

Soon it felt like everyone was against me. Even Averil, three years younger than me, was now more than my equal and was still keen to play the same rough and tumble games we had enjoyed before my operation. Whenever Rob or mum intervened – when the play escalated to full-scale warfare – Averil would complain bitterly at my preferential treatment. And, like my younger sister, Dorothy's amnesty on fighting ended once she was convinced I would not be going back to hospital anytime soon. As far as the girls were concerned, I was fair game. They only saw me as ill when I was lying prone on a hospital bed with tubes sticking out of me.

It all got too much for me and I demonstrated my misery in new nocturnal habits.

By now, some months into my sleep disorder, I was given my own room, possibly because no one could stomach being near me. Often mum would come in, just before she was going to bed, to find half my belongings lying on the lawn; I had thrown everything out of the window. Other times I would simply scream in fury and frustration, shouting for my dinner, even though I had just swallowed the last mouthful.

Ironically, although I found it impossible to sleep at night, I was still crippled by tiredness during the day. I had been back at school for several months now but the full days continued to take a lot out of me. While the other girls would return home from school, toss their bag into a corner and dash back out again to join their friends, I hung around the house and slept during the afternoon with my teddy bear.

The consequences of missing so much time off school were that my friends had settled into new routines with different chums. Often I would find myself at a loose end. Occasionally, mum's friend Hazel allowed me to go into her whisky shop on Fife Street in the afternoon. For 50 pence spending money, Hazel let me work in the shop, giving me a little tartan apron to wear. I think I was more a hindrance than a help because, grateful for the company, I would pester the customers with my idle chatter.

I began telling people about my tumour, giving them updates on my condition. Since I had come home from hospital, people had been genuinely worried about my chances of survival. Back then I was surprised anyone would want to take an interest in my situation. Now, back on my feet, I wanted to keep talking about my health.

It is the nature of towns like Dufftown that everyone quickly knows everyone else's business. Gossip spreads like wildfire and, once a story is out there, certain people feverishly await juicy updates. I decided to give them what I thought they wanted. Quite happy to discuss my on-going health saga, I would chat away about the medical implications of my predicament, sparing nothing as I told anyone who would listen, the gory details of my operations.

Despite this newfound openness, I was selective about what revelations I divulged. Secretly ashamed of my sleeping problems, I kept those incidents close to my chest. I did not want the local townsfolk whispering about the after dark nightmares in the Macdonald household.

And yet, even though I was tormented by guilt at what I was putting the family through, I was not able to conjure up a miracle cure to my insecurities.

Of course, mum tried to get to the bottom of my problems. She was forever taking me back to our beleaguered Dr Heneghan or driving me through to see the consultant paediatrician in Aberdeen. Mum was convinced my problems stemmed from the removal of the pineal gland, coupled with my anxiety over the tumour and my fear I might follow a similar fate to Caroline Nicol.

Apparently it has been documented that patients of pineal tumours have complained of irregular sleep patterns. Our consultants accepted my body clock could have been knocked out of kilter but they were at a loss to explain my odd pathological problems.

I had a simpler explanation. During one pow-wow with Mr Blaiklock in Aberdeen, I accused him of removing the "sleepy part of my head", when he was inside my brain. Mum then believed prescribing me melatonin might go some way to remedying my insomnia. She had read that businessmen in America take the drug to ward off the symptoms of jet lag and she knew the pineal gland is a natural source of melatonin in the body. Since my gland was removed it was reasonable to think that my body was being deprived of this substance. However, when she put this theory to a specialist in Aberdeen, he bluntly told her, "I take it you just want a social life?"

Mum was almost in tears. "I just want some sleep," she cried. "Three hours would be nice."

Desperately trying to find a rational explanation for my bizarre moods, she then also quizzed the specialists about the effects of Seasonal Affective Disorder (or SAD). She suggested the long, dark Scottish winters might be playing tricks on my sleep patterns. Research into SAD sufferers had concluded that people deprived of sunlight displayed symptoms more closely associated with depression. People waking up and coming home in darkness felt suicidal during the winter months, as their bodies adjusted to life without sun.

In a desperate bid to give us all some rest I was even prescribed adult-strength temazepam, or sleeping pills. The first time I took them they knocked me out for seven hours. I am sure the rest of the family would have been begging me to continue taking them but, sadly, the maximum dose was only twice a week. One night Dr Heneghan even came down to the house himself with sedation for me but at 2am he had to admit defeat because I was still awake. Mum was nearly at her wits' end.

The doctor offered her sleeping tablets but she refused. "I can sleep fine," she replied. "If I ever got the chance." Rob, though, did take the pills. Working the hours he did, he was desperate for some rest.

I had a life and, for that, I was grateful but the one I was now left with filled me with despair. As I neared the end of primary school, I was no closer to knowing what the future would hold. Two years after the operation to remove the first tumour, this was now my life; clinging to my parents and doing anything to stop sleeping in case I never woke up.

Chapter Thirteen
My Two Dads

Ever since I can remember, I have looked on Rob as my dad. Not being able to remember any time I lived with Archie on Skye before the split, I had nothing and no one to compare him to.

It must have been difficult for Archie to accept, but he knew I could not have been in better hands. Rob was as caring a man as you could ever meet – someone who would take a bullet for you. When he and mum got together there was never any doubt that he would step up to the plate and raise us as his children.

During my stays in hospital, Rob would sit by the bed until I fell asleep. With mum, he was the last person I saw before I was put to sleep; often he was the first person I saw when I regained my sight.

His dedication to his children was unquestionable. And, throughout my period of insomnia, he never complained.

Amazingly, despite my lack of sleep – I had been averaging about three hours a night every day for over a year now – I was displaying no real ill-effects. Sadly, the same cannot be said for Rob and the rest of my weary family, whose nerves were shredded.

I was often tired in the afternoon, once I returned home from school. The paediatrician suggested I needed a hobby or activity to occupy some brain cells and take my mind off my anxieties relating to the tumour. She thought if I was busy reading, or knitting, at night while the others were sleeping, it might take my mind off what was troubling me. It was easy for her to say. Mum and this particular consultant, to whom I had been visiting as an outpatient since my tumour operation, rarely saw eye-to-eye and frequently clashed on what was considered best for my development. Mum believed the doctor simply saw my situation in black and white and – because I did not display the textbook signs of brain damage – she filed my behavioural quirks into the drawer marked 'All in the mind'.

In fact, the doctor, a neurological paediatrician, went further and even suggested the sleeplessness was a by-product of poor parenting. As you can imagine, clinical assessments like that did not go down well with mum, who, from the moment I became ill, was never anything other than completely committed to my well-being. It seemed clear to mum I was experiencing severe psychological trauma.

Nobody, who has not experienced what it is like to live with a tumour, can really say what effect it has on a patient.

Finally, the specialist relented and referred me to a psychiatrist, who was to get results but not in the areas we would have first thought.

In the sessions, which I would attend with mum, the female doctor explored the effects the tumour was having on my emotional state. We examined the impact Caroline's death was having on me and she explained that my friend's situation, although on the surface remarkably similar, was hugely different. I was seeing our fates inextricably linked. I could see no outcome other than the one set out for her. The way I saw it, I had a tumour in my head that the surgeons could not take out. They were not able to take out the one in my friend's head and I saw what happened to her. However, the doctor tried to explain that I was seeing the world in child-like terms, which was hard for me to take. After all, I was a child! She explained there was a mountain of reasons why my life should not be compared to anyone else's. I had lots to live for, she stressed.

Instead, she explored the possibility my problems could stem from friction inside our family. As she took us down that particular path, she asked me about my relationships with other members of the family. Before we knew it, Pandora's Box was blown open and we were discussing all the intricate dynamics in the house. I confessed it was confusing growing up not knowing really who my dad was. I mean, I knew. The problem was that now even Averil, after Dorothy and Robina, was challenging my right to call him dad.

It was hard, I said, to know my place in the house. Dorothy knew her dad, Robina certainly knew because she lived with him and now Averil was safe and secure in the knowledge of her parentage.

As a result of these revelations, the doctor summoned the rest of the family to add their opinions. But the girls, faced with a strange inquisitor and unsure what the implications were, clammed up. However, the sessions with the shrink got mum and dad thinking.

Shortly after our last meeting, mum and Rob sat me down. How would I like Rob to adopt me, they asked.

Until that point, I had never considered the thought. In my heart I knew he was my dad. I did not see why it needed a bit of paper to make it official. Their reasons made perfect sense though. My future was uncertain and I might require further surgery on my head. Up until that point mum, as my main legal guardian, had to sign-off all the consent forms for operations. With Rob formally recognised as my father, mum would not need to be there all the time. In addition, it would make it easier in the house. He would legally be my dad. It would be official. I would take the name Macdonald.

There was one small problem. How would I tell my real dad?

Dorothy was holidaying in Skye at Archie's when the decision was made to break the news to him. Mum called him first. She explained the reasons why Rob should adopt me. Archie initially objected. He could not see the need to have a formal adoption.

Then, it was time for me to speak. I remember coming on the phone and saying firmly: "I want Rob to be my dad."

Archie didn't know what to say. He knew he had little emotional credit in the bank where I was concerned. I had left home when I was eighteen months old. This didn't make it any easier for him though.

Dorothy and Robina looked on as, once the call ended, Archie took himself to the bathroom and wept, almost sick with sorrow. I had no idea at the time how this affected him. To me, it seemed a simple decision, a transfer of dads.

To his credit though, Archie did not contest the decision. I would not have had the strength if my dads had started fighting over me, especially with all my associated health problems.

And so, in August 1992, I officially became Caroline Macdonald. It was the best £400 my new dad Rob ever spent.

79

It wouldn't be the only change in the house. Dorothy, although not formally adopted, would also take dad's name. It wasn't much but the simple act held a huge significance for me. Suddenly it felt like we were a normal family.

Yet, while the adoption granted me the security I craved, it failed to steady my night-time panic attacks.

Even the theories of the paediatrician, although well intentioned, had little impact. I did take her advice on board, however. I was already interested in needlework after picking it up at primary school so I chose to try my hand at knitting. Mum had a knitting machine at home. For years she had been churning out mohair cardigans for us all, that made us itch so much it looked like we were all infested with fleas.

Before long I was churning out my own creations. The knitting would have worked wonders if there had suddenly been a worldwide kitchen cloth shortage, but it did nothing for my restlessness at night.

In general terms, my health picked up though. The headaches, which had become my signature trait, subsided for a while and I enjoyed an unbroken period at school, my first for a long time. Soon, though, I was finding I had the run of the place. Teachers believed the best course of action, and who could blame them, was to wrap me in cotton wool almost to the extent that I had been in hospital. They did not have much experience of dealing with children with tumours. Regularly I nodded off in class and was allowed to do so. My schoolwork suffered and it really became noticeable when Averil started catching up on me, despite the three-year age gap.

In an attempt to give the family some respite, mum employed the services of Crossroads nurses, a charity that supply volunteers to help ease the workload on overburdened families. On several occasions, once a month, a woman would come to the house in the evening and sit up to allow everyone else to go to bed. Then, when I rose in the middle of the night, there would be someone there to deal with my moods. I would sit up talking with these kindly souls; it gave me reassurance that someone was on standby, a little like it had been when I was in hospital.

Another person who provided valuable respite care and moral support was Kenny Ferguson of the MacMillan Nurses, a charity offering care and support to the families of cancer sufferers. One afternoon a week, he would pop into the house and talk through our situation during these tormented days. Mum was grateful for his support. No one had a miracle cure for what ailed me but he sympathised with my mum in her quest for finding some explanation for my irrational behaviour.

Many times since, I've tried to find reason in my own mind as to why I behaved in such a manner.

I craved mum's full attention even though I had been receiving it for years. I accept I was demanding and put my parents and sisters through hell, but I still believe no one can judge me. All I ask is that they put themselves in my place for just one day to see how they would react to a similar situation. Part of it was down to the surgery, part of it was the length of time I had spent in hospital, part of it was the fear that I was going to die and part of it was that the attention I received at home spoiled me. Sometimes, my family treated me like royalty, lifts to school while my classmates walked, excused from even the most menial tasks and being showered with gifts.

None of the people who judged me knew what I was going through. They didn't know what it was like for me. You cannot begin to imagine what I was thinking at night, the demons that haunted me and the horrors filling my head. I would not wish any child to have to go through what I endured. I thought about the tumour all the time. I wondered why surgeons could not remove it. I wondered why I could not get chemotherapy or radiotherapy. Neither was an option for me. When I was in hospital I saw children around me receiving this treatment and thought of it eating away at their tumours, while mine just grew and grew. Radiotherapy, too, was an option for some children, but considered too risky for me.

Hospital is a horrible place for a child to be. I probably did not appreciate it at the time but, subconsciously, seeing and hearing the children around me with their terrible diseases had an impact on me.

Irrespective of this, I felt safe in hospital because, in that environment, I had doctors and nurses on call around me to take care of my every whim. Most of the time mum was with me and I did not have to share her with the other children. Mum was in hospital with me; she was part of the team.

Then, when I came home, with the tumour still lodged in my brain, I did not feel safe. In the house, nobody watched over me while I slept. Worst of all, at home, I had to share mum with the other children. And since I had been back full time at home, I was still confused about my place in the house. From being an assertive young girl, I felt weakened; physically by the tumour and emotionally as I felt my histrionics were to blame for the family's stresses. At the time there was a lot of conflict in the house, probably because everyone was walking on a knife-edge, their nerves shattered through lack of sleep, worrying what I would come up with next.

For that I felt responsible. I wanted to be a better child for mum. I just could not help the way I was though.

I think, at this point in time, no one believed I could get any worse. Not for the first time, I proved them wrong.

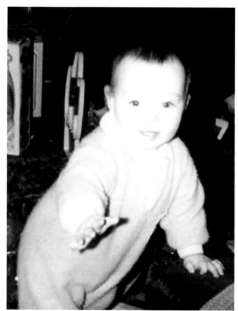

Taking my first steps as a toddler.

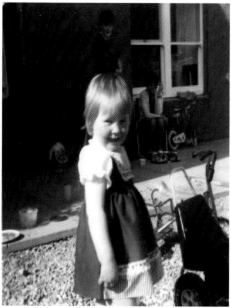

Me, aged 3, shortly before my world was turned upside down.

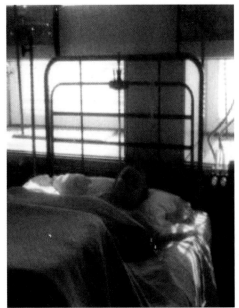

Feeling groggy after my first op.

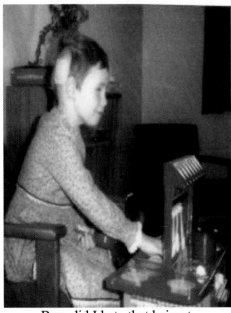

Boy, did I hate that haircut.

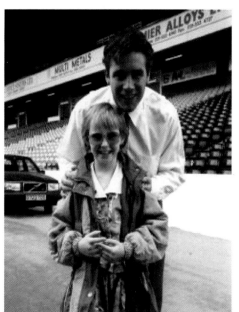

Ally McCoist with Elton John. Oops, sorry, that's me!

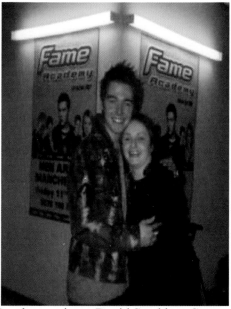

Fame Academy winner David Sneddon. Gets my vote!

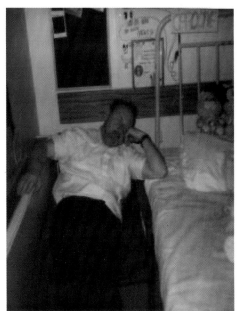

Here's Rob, sleeping on the job.

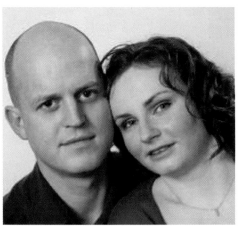

Me, with the man of my dreams.

Chapter Fourteen
A New Danger

New Year was always a bittersweet time for mum. Every Hogmanay, as she nursed a tipple before the bells she would stand by the patio doors which led out to the front garden and tears would well in her eyes.

Ever since I became sick with hydrocephalus and her father developed heart problems, she had started this little ritual. She never confided in us why this was but I like to think it was for two reasons; she was sorrowful for the suffering we had both endured but was glad that we had made it through another year.

The night that heralded the dawn of 1993 was no exception. I wonder if, as she gazed to the stars, she pondered what lay in store for her beloved family that, by then, had suffered more than its fair share of grief. If so, she would not have to wait long for her answer.

On 2nd January, mum planned a fun-filled start to the New Year. We were going ice-skating with Dr Heneghan, his family and some friends. Shortly before we were due to leave, I was watching television, rewinding a video. At the time, Rob was standing in the kitchen waiting, as he always did, for the kids to get their stuff together.

Then it happened.

At first mum thought this was it. My time had come. All she could see was me, lying prone on the floor, jerking uncontrollably, my eyes thrown back in my head. She grabbed the phone and dialled the doctor's number from memory.

"Come quickly," she begged. She did not need to say who she was or give her address. The doc knew only too well where to come.

I was having my first epileptic seizure; a grand mal.

What had triggered it was the video rewinding – the shaky images on screen were too much for the mind to comprehend, sparking a lightening storm in my brain.

The seizure was over in moments. Of course, when I came to I had no recollection of what had happened, just a hazy feeling in my head and grogginess I normally associated with my operations.

In the immediate aftermath, it meant yet more examinations. The surgeons were not surprised. Apparently epilepsy is a common side affect of brain surgery, although everyone could have a seizure if given adequate stimulus. When the surgeons fitted my original shunt, the trauma on my brain could have been enough to trigger it. Alternatively the tumour itself may have brought it on. Either way it was yet another thing for me to contend with.

My doctor put me on medication to control the seizures and, although this seemed to control the attacks, I subsequently started to feel chronic pins and needles in my arms at night that kept me awake – as if I needed that.

I wish I could say that, when medics confirmed the epilepsy, I took it in my stride and strove to overcome it. The truth is far removed from that. I took it badly and started to believe I was cursed. I could not understand why this was happening to me. Already with enough hang-ups to single me out from my schoolmates, I did not need another. Not for the first time, I began to feel sorry for myself.

Doctors tried to lift my spirits by saying I was in esteemed company. Bud Abbott of Abbott and Costello fame turned to drink to hide his epilepsy, the Lethal Weapon actor Danny Glover learned to live with his for 20 years and Young One star, Rik Mayall, suffered two seizures after failing to take his medication. Little comfort for an eleven-year-old girl.

Thankfully, medication restricted the grand mals, or full-scale convulsions, to a minimum, but I did not escape the petit mals, or panic attacks. In many ways I found these more terrifying because I was aware of them happening. For just a few seconds my body would shut down and, although I could hear the concerned voices around me, I was powerless to react, as if paralysed in my own private hell. They would come on without warning, striking me when I least expected it. All I could do was sit there, gasping for breath, waiting for the moment to pass, wondering if I would choke to death.

Given what I had been through, I might have been expected to cope with the new challenge but I saw it simply as a horrifying addition to an already troubled existence.

My mother, sensing the trouble I was in, feared the move to secondary school, awaiting me in just four months, was beyond me at this stage. With dad, she met with my teachers, who agreed the best course of action was to stay on at Mortlach Primary and repeat my final year.

It made perfect sense. After surgeons fitted the shunt, I missed virtually all of Primary Two, crucial in the development of any small child. Then, when they found the tumour, I missed another huge portion of schooling. Mum feared my classmates would leave me further behind and worried what such feelings of failure would do to me. In hindsight, mum wishes she had brought in a tutor to teach me at home but she was so desperate for me to rejoin the other children and wanted so much for me to have a normal life where I could mingle with other children my age. Plus, because I started school aged only four, effectively I would be still be the same age as the people in my year when I was kept back.

Yes, it made perfect sense; except to me.

The last thing I wanted was anything else that drew attention to my plight. It was bad enough that I was receiving remedial teaching in an attempt to stay in touch with my peers. Now I was to suffer the indignity of being kept back. Children, in those situations, do not see brain tumours, or operations; they see "thickos".

I watched as my friends left school and moved on without me, while I was stuck with the younger kids. I struggled to accept this arrangement and I must have been a handful for my Primary Seven teacher as I sat sulking at the back of the class for the whole year.

Throughout this time, the neurosurgeons were still monitoring my tumour through six-monthly scans. It was growing but not significantly enough to cause them great concern, they said. What they *were* worried about was my continued lack of growth. As children, we progress at different rates but, as I prepared for high school, it was now noticeable that I was lagging behind, not just educationally but also physically. My mother was fairly tall and, although my dad was not exceptionally so, he came from a large family. Dorothy was tall and slim and Averil was now almost as big as I was.

I seemed to be forever being sent for tests; I had tests on bones, tests on my thyroid, and tests of my growth hormones. I was even tested for oestrogen, as the medics feared the operations had affected my sexual development. A clean bill of health was never going to be on the cards but I could have done with just a glimpse of a silver lining on the storm of dark clouds over my head.

It was not forthcoming. Instead, in the next few weeks, inexplicably, I lost my sense of balance and, almost overnight, forgot how to ride a bicycle. Suffering from a lack of co-ordination since my tumour operation, I lost certain skills I had learned as a child. What is it they say? You never forget how to ride a bike. So, in the same way nurses had to teach me to walk again, it seemed that I would need a refresher course if I was ever to get back in the saddle. We all had bikes at Scorrybreck, even mum and dad, and whenever possible we would go for cycle rides along the Speyside Way, a popular walking route along the river that gives the region its name.

Once I started to regain my strength I was looking forward to going back out on two wheels. However, as soon as I climbed on the saddle, it was clear I was not going to be able to pick up where I left off. As my mountain bike started to wobble off down the drive to the main road, I could not understand why such a simple thing was proving so difficult. I was like a shopping trolley with a wonky wheel. Every time I set off, the bike veered over to one side and ditched me at the side of the road.

I've since rediscovered the knack of riding a bike but sometimes I still suffer problems. During one of the last times I went out, with Robina, I mastered the art of peddling up hills yet curiously could only push the bike downhill.

The setback was not serious in the grand scheme of things but it was yet another example of something other children did in their sleep that was suddenly beyond me.

In addition, I was preparing to make the leap to high school and, although I had resented repeating Primary Seven, I was not convinced I was ready for the challenges awaiting me.

Chapter Fifteen
Little Miss Nobody

Speyside High School sits only seven miles away from Dufftown, in Aberlour, but it could have been on another planet as far as I was concerned.

I resented repeating my final year at primary school and spent my time moping at the rear of the classroom, cursing my luck and wishing the days away until I could take my place at the big school. When the time came for my first day, I was dreading the step up.

I was relieved I would be joining Dorothy but the prospect of catching the morning bus was very different from the leisurely walk I previously enjoyed to the village school.

What I did not realise was that, for my big sister, my presence at her school was about as welcome as the proverbial number two in a swimming pool. The last role she wanted was as babysitter to her troublesome little sister. No sooner had we jumped on the school bus than she bounced off to join her friends, leaving me to make conversation with the conductor down at the front.

It was a mere taste of things to come.

For days, I followed her about like a newborn duckling at break-times, oblivious to her signals that I was cramping her style. Grateful for any scraps of attention she and her friends would throw me, I developed a thick skin to their teasing, telling myself I was one of the gang.

The problem was, because of the extra time I had spent in primary school, the age gap between us had now effectively stretched to four years – practically a generation in teen years.

Who could blame her? After the grief she had put up with at home, it was a wonder she even gave me the time of day.

At first, I tried anything to get her attention. If she were hanging out with her friends when I went up to her, she would cringe as I approached. That might have had something to do with that fact I hollered "Yoo-ee", in a glass-shattering voice from across the playground. (I still do to this day!) Although she would make it perfectly clear my company was not wanted, I desperately longed to hang out with her and her friends, and would try anything for a reaction. Unfortunately, the only purpose I seemed to serve was as the butt of their jokes, but it almost did not matter.

I was trying so hard to be accepted but I was loud and brash and craving attention. I began bugging Dorothy so much she tripped me up in the corridor one afternoon, sending me sprawling on the floor. Acting as if I had been shot, I writhed on the ground, clutching my leg as if it was broken. Despite my tumour, Dorothy saw me just like any other little sister – well, any sister who kept their elder siblings awake half the night, stole their duvet covers and half their clothes and sat up in bed shouting.

Trying to keep up with Dot was not my only concern. The hectic pace of the new school stunned me. From sharing Mortlach with some 160 other kids, I was now one solitary figure amidst nearly 600 hulking bodies, each one twice the size of me, it seemed.

Used to setting my toys and trinkets around my desk at primary school for the last eight years, here I had to gather my belongings, and hurry along the corridors, up and down stairs, for the next lesson. The school day just seemed to be a succession of sprint races to see who could get to the next class first.

Immediately, I was out of my depth. Blessed with the concentration span of a goldfish, I struggled to keep up with the pace of higher education. By the time I finally twigged which class I was in, it was time to move on to the next lesson. Moreover, with all the extra subjects, it seemed the teachers were speaking in a foreign language. They babbled at me like the schoolmistresses in Charlie Brown, barking alien concepts in monotone, directing me to textbooks written in Sanskrit. In desperation, I started copying from my classmates, straining my neck to see over their shoulders. It worked, for a nanosecond or until Sir asked me how I arrived at a particular answer. Then, for the first time in my life, I felt sensations of flushing to the face, which I could not blame on the tumour. Quickly, I was realising I did suffer from a brain defect – an inability to learn. I felt like a dunce, hopelessly out of my depth.

On a social level, I was equally at sea. It was an eternal source of frustration for me that there were so many children, yet no one with whom I could speak. People seemed to be so busy with their own lives and friends. It didn't help that my old classmates from Mortlach were a year ahead and, in accordance with teenager law, forbade conversation with a child in the year below. In addition, the people with whom I made the jump to high school saw me as an outsider, someone considered too old for their class, even though I shared birthdays with them.

To make matters worse, back then I was a slip of a girl who was forced to wear geeky-looking standard issue National Health Service specs. Invariably, I would snap the legs off them and be forced to patch them up with sticky tape, looking like a junior Jack Duckworth from Coronation Street.

At break times, I walked around by myself; little Miss Nobody. I was so lonely I resorted to hanging around with the janitor in the tuck shop. If other children raised their eyebrows at my presence behind the counter, I told them I was only helping restock shelves. I tried to convince myself that was the case; rather than face the truth; that he was the only person in school who would speak to me. I remember, having no one to talk to or hang about with, walking around the school grounds myself like a weirdo. Alternatively, I would duck into the library and pretend to read or try to catch up with my work, which I always found too hard to do in class and never had enough time to finish. It got me down that none of the children took the time to get to know me or let me join in their groups.

Eventually, two girls did make an effort to involve me in their activities. Jennifer and Caitlin, from Aberlour and Ballindalloch respectively, were in my class almost from the start. Unlike the other kids, they accepted me for who I was. Mostly the rest had no idea how to handle me. They tiptoed around me either because of my tumour or because my newfound directness unnerved them. Both girls were normal teenagers. They were obsessed with their hair but, while they would sit for the whole of break preening, I would look in the mirror wondering what they found to fuss about. Still, I cannot deny that I was grateful for the attention. They were quite pretty and attracted lots of interest from boys but, sadly, none of the attention rubbed off on me and, for the most part, I was in a twilight zone, stalking the corridors like a ghost.

It hurt me to see how popular Dorothy was and then, when Averil came up to the school, that she was too. That made things worse. Sometimes I was so miserable I pretended I had a sore head so I could go and lie in the medical room.

One day I stunned everyone in my class by taking a panic attack right in the middle of a music tutorial. I remember being frozen with fear and, terrified, I hid under the table until the episode passed.

However, with that situation, I began to realise that, as in primary school, I was something of a novelty. Once again, mine was the only brain tumour in class. Word had spread about the operations and people eyed me up like a science exhibit. Was my head going to pop at any moment? Was the tumour like a second head? That's what I imagined they were thinking. At first, it unnerved me, being the focus of curiosity but fairly soon I began to relish the notoriety and used it to my advantage.

The more I fell behind in class, the greater the pressure I was under to keep up. At first, the stress brought on the old symptoms – dizziness, tiredness and headaches. The response was predictable. At the first sign of trouble, teachers packed me off to the sickbay. From there, either the nurse allowed me to recuperate or mum would get the call to come and take me home.

If mum ever believed starting secondary school would signal a fresh start for her daughter, she was sorely mistaken. Near the end of the first year, when she went to the annual Parents' Evening, conversations with two of my eight teachers were enough to convince her otherwise. After that, she had heard enough. She collared my guidance teacher.

"This is the first Parents' Night I have been to for Caroline at high school and it will be the last," she said bluntly. "It's not that I take issue with what the teachers are saying. Everything they say is true. I just don't need to hear what I already know."

It became clear that many of the teachers, and pupils, were inexperienced when it came to dealing with children who had

91

serious neurological issues; not that they had much choice of course. Faced with that situation, how many teachers would set aside their instinct that perhaps the child was exaggerating the incident? Not only did I have a tumour, but I was also epileptic and lived with a tube in my neck. No teacher wanted me to pass out on his or her watch.

I am not proud to say this, but soon I started to realise I could take advantage of the situation. Whenever I felt the lesson was too difficult, on would come a headache. Not confident of passing a surprise test? Dizzy spell will fix that. Alternatively, if I had forgotten my homework for the last lesson of the day, I would suddenly succumb to a bout of chronic fatigue. It is shameful, I know and, looking back, I cringe at the thought of taking my teachers' goodwill for granted.

Gradually, seeing I was getting away with it, I became more of a handful for my teachers. I used to complain all the time. I would forever be moaning of headaches and not feeling well. It was easy.

For one French reading exam, I took one look at the paper, stuck up my hand and said: "Sorry. I'm not feeling well." I got out of the exam.

Looking back, I realise that all too easily I accepted that my illness gave me an excuse not to buckle down in class. I had no inclination to do well. If I were to do it all over again I would definitely work a lot harder. I regret my behaviour at school.

The teachers did not know how to handle me. I think they were scared to treat me as harshly as they treated other kids because they were afraid of my condition. They tiptoed around me in the early years, fearful of what an ear bashing might do to me. I used to get away with murder. Moreover, if I did not get what I wanted, I used to walk out of class. In many ways, it was shocking that they allowed me to get away with it.

Some days, I would not even make it to school. In the morning, if I suspected a heavy day lay ahead, I just had to say to mum I had a headache and she would say, 'Okay'. It was a terrible way to treat mum, showing a complete lack of respect for what she had sacrificed for me. However, when you are thirteen you only see life through the eyes of a teenager, and believe the world exists for your benefit.

Now I wish everyone had been more forceful and had the courage to act only when they suspected something was seriously wrong.

At the time, I believed I was so clever. Chuckling at the gullibility of my teachers, I thought they were the mugs for falling for my charades.

Now I see that I was the mug.

In the long term, my reluctance to apply myself harmed only me. I am still paying for my actions today. If I could turn back the clock and, instead of languishing in the sickbay, knuckled down and concentrated harder perhaps I could have performed better at school.

Often, while attending Aberdeen Royal Infirmary for my three monthly check-ups as an outpatient I even had the cheek to criticise the staff at Speyside, accusing them of molly-coddling me and failing to knock me into shape.

I cannot blame the teachers for how they handled me. It must have been a difficult position for them. I am only lucky I did not pay for crying wolf and I'm thankful my selfishness spared me a serious episode.

Nevertheless, it is always easy to look back with hindsight. At the time, I felt much maligned. I felt miserable at school and, up until I was fourteen, struggled to make much of an impact.

At home, I was still in a terrible state at night, looking for someone to sit up with me through the twilight hours.

In my despair, I could see no way out of this misery. I tried to run away several times, but even at something as easy as this, I failed. Once, I packed a suitcase with all my worldly belongings, threw it out of the window and clambered out after it. My disappearance was noticed immediately – probably because, for once, there was silence in my room. Rob rushed out into the street looking for me and, after less than an hour, found me standing on the main road, near the Glenfiddich distillery, some two hundred yards from the house.

It was a miserable attempt to shock my parents. It wasn't their fault I was so depressed. They were only doing what they thought was right. Still, I felt I had missed out so much on the simple things other children take for granted. While Dorothy and Averil nipped out to spend the night at a friend's sleepover,

I rarely went anywhere without mum and dad. Even on our trips to Skye, I would remain under the watchful eye of my parents, while Dorothy lived it up with Archie and Robina, I imagined, having a far better time than I was.

Mum, by this point, though, had suffered enough. I do not think any mother could imagine what it must have been like for her. She tried everything to make me better. Then, when there were no longer any viable solutions, she took radical action. Instead of my feeble attempts to shock her, it was her turn to stun me.

In February 1996, when I was fourteen, my parents put me into care.

Chapter Sixteen
In Exile

I think that to understand what makes a mother send her child away from home you would have to have spent a night in our house.

Mum was at the end of her tether. All the theories she had explored, the support she had sought and the solutions she had tried were fruitless.

The more she tried to soothe my insecurities and calm my fears, the clingier I became. Feeling isolated by health professionals who scoffed at the seriousness of the situation, she was at a loss how to save not only her sanity but also that of the family.

Dr Heneghan sympathised with her plight. Standing by us through thick and thin, he had seen mum teeter on the brink of despair with the hydrocephalus and then the tumour. Each time she had prepared for the worst. And, although in every case she had found salvation, a new crisis was waiting just round the corner.

Through it all, however, our local GP stepped up to the plate. He was the rock mum relied on through all her travails and he could tell how much she needed respite from her troublesome daughter. I am ashamed to admit it now, but I was suffocating the life out of our family. Despite all that, it was still with a heavy heart he recommended to mum a charity set up to help parents in exactly her situation.

Aberlour Child Care Trust was an organisation that owed its origins to an orphanage, which opened its doors in 1875, offering much-needed shelter to "motherless bairns". Miss MacPherson Grant, who, with the support of chaplain Canon Charles Jupp, founded the trust; launching a church, school and orphanage in the town's Burnside Cottage. They held the belief, though unpopular at the time, that every child had the ability to grow up and blossom in society, regardless of their heritage or economic status. Canon Jupp worked tirelessly, preaching and appealing for funds and started an annual jumble sale to keep the project afloat. Today, the trust thrives, providing help and support to families of children from all backgrounds.

Among its projects throughout Morayshire was Alba Place, a two-tiered centre in Elgin that principally offered long-term residential care for children with profound learning disabilities. However, it was the second arm to the project – providing short-break respite care for parents and children suffering from a wide range of disabilities – which our doctor thought might offer mum a beacon of hope in her maelstrom of despair.

At first the suggestion appalled her. She could never send her child away. It would seem like banishing me for being imperfect, in the way nineteenth century society dealt with its problems. Then children, who were born out of wedlock or were discovered to have profound mental or physical disabilities, were exiled from the family unit. They were doomed to live out their days in an orphanage, poor house or a church home run by strict disciplinarian nuns.

Mum was adamant. Yes, I was a problem. Anyone who spent five minutes in our house of an evening would testify to that but foisting me off on strangers? That was not the answer. There had to be an alternative.

Confiding in friends and relatives, she broached the subject of the respite care. Could they believe what she was being asked to do, she said. How was a mother to live with the decision that she had finally thrown in the towel? Putting me into care would be like admitting defeat – like announcing she, my mother, was no longer prepared to deal with the sleepless nights. It would be someone else's problem. After all we had been through, she had finally reached breaking point. What signal would that send to the other children; that, if they pushed her far enough, they too would be out the door? What kind of mother would behave like that towards her own flesh and blood?

The response she received, though, from her trusted loved ones took her by surprise.

Take a step back from her life, they urged. She needed a dose of perspective. As things were, the family were hostages to my psychotic episodes. Normal people cannot function on only three hours of sleep a night. The longer this torment continued, the bigger the strain it would put on the family. Relationships, already stretched to breaking point, would disintegrate. It was that serious. Radical problems called for radical solutions. Imagine the luxury of a guaranteed full night's sleep, three days a week? A chance to recharge the batteries, recapture some semblance of your normal life; a life lost to a tragic catalogue of medical misery. How much better equipped would she be to deal with my condition and its associated problems? She would be re-energised and rejuvenated for the fight, ready once again to tackle whichever trauma was next sent to try us.

It would not be for eternity – just two or three nights a week. The change of scene might do me good and make me realise there were people far worse off than myself. The reality check might shake me from whatever it was that was keeping me awake during the dark nights.

Reluctantly mum knew everyone was right. She was on her last legs. Previously strong enough to soak up any situation thrown at the family, she was now effectively at the end of her tether. If she didn't act now, how would she be able to react if something should befall any of her other children? Until this point she had been lucky. Robina, Dorothy and Averil had got on with the job of living relatively stress-free. Would that always be the case? My history had taught her many things; not least that she could not afford to take things for granted. Plus, many parents took advantage of respite care offered to them. It was a vital support system enabling them to continue devoting love and care to their beloved offspring.

So it was, still with a sense of guilt lying heavy on her conscience, she took the first steps to put me into care.

A single-storey building set in its own grounds on the northern outskirts of Elgin; Alba House was a first class facility for people living with disabilities. Boasting long-term accomodation for six children and short-term stay for several others, the trust treated each resident to their own private room, with shared toilet and bathroom facilities and living quarters.

Staff advised my parents to bring me to the home, to see the accommodation and acclimatise to the surroundings before committing me to my first overnight stay.

Mum tried to convince me I would like it. It would be like it was in Aberdeen Royal Infirmary, she said, a place I had felt secure and safe; where, at night, someone was always awake to watch over me as I slept. Of course, mum would not be there but the support network I apparently craved would.

Despite the sales pitch, my first impressions were not favourable. To me, a teenage girl, I only thought cruel things about the place. In my mind, I mistakenly believed I had the home sussed in seconds. It was a child prison, a funny farm for problem kids. Now, I can accept the reasons for putting me there. Then, though, my objections were not a consideration. I was going, like it or not.

It was agreed that I would arrive, once a month, on Friday nights and stay for three nights, travelling straight to school on Monday morning from Elgin.

I would not have admitted it at the time, but the carers were first class. Friendly and professional, they did everything possible to make the centre a home for the children there. Dealing mostly with youngsters with Down's syndrome, cerebral palsy and other physically and mentally challenged kids, they were expert at improving the lives of their charges who responded with joy to the attention lavished upon them.

The experience I have of seeing children, some the same age as me, taking the most out of life, despite the cruel hand dealt to them, affected me profoundly. The trouble was it took me several years for the positives from my time there to register in my brain. I cherish the time I spent in Alba House and I am grateful my situation, however precarious, still allows me to live a full and happy life.

However, like I said, my attitude now contrasts sharply with my reasoning then. Why was I here, I thought? I was nothing like these children, who couldn't even hold a conversation with me. Once again, I was cursed. Misunderstood and persecuted, this was surely just another episode in my general drama of misery. Was there no way out of this torment?

Lying in my bed at night, with only a few personal keepsakes around me for comfort, I slated my supposed family who put me here. They would be out enjoying themselves, living it up, going to the cinema, the pub, out with friends, laughing about how happy they were now Caroline was out of the picture. I was a leper, cast out from my own community.

They would all be laughing at me, hoping the short, sharp shock treatment, would rewire my brain and turn me back into a normal, happy child. Why would no one believe me? Even my mum, my saviour in times of trouble, had turned her back on me. And dad, the one who had raised me as his own and loved me more than any natural father could, had done nothing to stop this. Curse them all, I thought.

I was sickeningly dismissive of my fellow residents, wrongly convinced I was superior to them. For entertainment, carers took me to the cinema with some of the other children but I did not want to be seen in public with the group, worried people would think I was "one of them". Paranoid what the other children in the picture house would think of my party, I cruelly imagined them staring at me.

"I shouldn't be here," I wanted to shout.

I was judging people by my own prejudices, imagining others would be as condescending if the tables were turned and I came across a group of these children.

I am now ashamed of my attitude but then I blamed them for my problems. It was not anyone else's fault I was in a care home. It was mine, because I was not emotionally strong enough to realise I had been given a second chance in life. I failed to see I was the lucky one and could only conclude I was cursed by the tumour growing on my brain.

What made it worse was arriving at school on Monday mornings. Children pick up on anything different from the norm and, although no one said anything to my face, I was certain they would be gossiping behind my back – laughing at the "handicapped" kid arriving from the special needs care home. Arriving at the school by any other method than the bus from Dufftown only served to further fuel my paranoia that the other pupils were sniggering behind my back.

I wanted to fit, be one of the gang, and the last thing I needed was more reasons to be different.

Any initial improvement my weekend stays had on my sleep patterns was debatable. In fact, during my first couple of times away mum wondered if it was worth the effort. The sleep my carers promised her did not materialise, probably because I spent the first few nights awake and, with nothing better to do, I used whatever change I could lay my hands on to call the house … repeatedly.

Mum despaired. What was the point in paying a private health care home a small fortune if I was just going to find new methods of keeping her awake?

"I'm lonely," I would tell her at 2am. "What are you doing?"

"Trying to get some sleep," she replied. "Like I do most nights."

If the aim of this experiment was to let everyone get some sleep, I obviously had not read the script.

Still, though, they persevered. My visits increased to twice a month.

However, to everyone's surprise, not least my own, my behaviour gradually got a little better. Resigned to the situation, my attitude changed, ever so slightly. I would not go so far as saying I made the most of the experience, but I accepted the situation and, slowly, adapted to my temporary surroundings.

As one of the few children in the centre who could participate in every activity, I became more involved and, dare I admit it, started to enjoy myself. My carers encouraged me to help with the cooking and cleaning and I revelled in my new found responsibilities. I also warmed to the facilities and took great pleasure soaking in the huge spa bath in one of the communal bathrooms. Relaxing in the bubbles, I conceded this was far better than the bath we had back home. This place wasn't so bad, I admitted.

As I was more on a par with the carers than the other residents, I began to have the run of the place and enjoyed the freedom. Whether they thought it, I cannot say, but my nurse friends certainly never said if they thought my behaviour odd and I began to feel appreciated. The staff did not judge me and accepted me for who I was.

Yet, while I at least made some effort to tolerate the place, I still yearned to go home and, from the middle of the week before I was due to leave, dreaded the time it came for mum to drive me to Elgin.

Mercifully, the experiment only lasted a few months and mum and Rob accepted I was no better off at Alba House than at home.

It was a relief to be back at Scorrybreck once again but my time away had not significantly improved my ability to sleep through the night. Frustratingly, my behaviour was still full of contradictions. Tired and listless during the day, I was restless at night. Although my sleeplessness was not now a nightly occurrence, it was still a factor. Mostly I would go to bed at 9.30pm, lie awake for an hour and stir once or twice a night before getting up at 7am.

Following further consultations, the paediatricians in Aberdeen suggested prescribing diazepam sleeping tablets occasionally. The pills had some effect, although often it would take me until midnight to doze off, but I would sleep through to seven o'clock.

However, due to the addictive nature of such tablets, my doctors were reluctant to prescribe them on a regular basis. They offered me a mild anti-depressant in the hope the mild hypnotic qualities of the drug might knock me into a settled pattern. I refused. Even though by now, I was ready to try almost anything, the thought of turning into more of a zombie than I felt already did not hold much appeal.

It was now six years since surgeons discovered the tumour and I was about to enter my sixth year of sleepless nights.

Running out of suggestions, Dr Heneghan mentioned to mum that the local hospital in Dufftown also offered temporary respite care but mum, who regretted putting me through my Alba House experience, declined. She knew she could not live with herself if she sent me away again. She knew there would be no miracle solution. The strategy she had employed since day one – to soldier on praying things would get better – was the only available option.

Chapter Seventeen
We are Family

Blimey, what a misery fest you must think my life was. Who would want to live in a house with me?

While I am trying to give an accurate portrayal of what life was like for me as I struggled to come to terms with the awful realisation that I was living with an inoperable brain tumour, it would be wrong of me to suggest there were no moments of happiness for us.

There were.

Mostly they were restricted to when we were all away on holiday. I don't know what it was about being on vacation but it seemed to bring out the best in all of us. Maybe, in those two weeks, we were the same as any other family. Freed from the shackles of everyday life, jobs and school, we relaxed and remembered what we liked about each other.

Whatever the reason, it seemed that the only respite mum – and the rest of the family for that matter – received was during our annual breaks.

As far as I can remember, our vacations were the few times we could look back on with fond memories. My earliest memory of foreign travel was a trip to Spain when I was five and we were yet to be blighted by my health problems. The whole gang was there, including Michael. We stayed in a plush hotel. I recall my sisters and I spent most of our days in the children's club, much to mum and dad's delight, no doubt.

I'm sure mum and dad, as they walked on the sand in the evening, must have dreamed of many more sun-seeking trips. They were not to know the path events would take and that it would be five years before they would next get a break away from the troubles at home.

Several months after my tumour operation, and once the doctors had given me the all-clear to travel, we headed for Majorca with mum's friend, Helen Nixon, and her family. It was great to get away and catch some sun, although, typically I was horrendously sunburnt, with blisters popping out all over my arms.

After that trip, mum and dad were determined we had suffered enough and always tried to ensure that, whatever dramas were rocking us, we would at least try to enjoy two weeks away as a family.

So, the following year, we headed off once again to Majorca, to Palma Nova, with the Nixons. While the rest of the family had a great time, however, it was a strange time for me. While the others lay stretched out on their sunloungers, soaking up the warm Mediterranean rays, I was lost under a mountain of towels on the beach. While I might have been able to get more rest in the balmy foreign climate, my internal temperature gauge was all to pot. It might have been thirty degrees outside but I was shivering. As the rest stripped to their bathing costumes and trunks, I was decked out head to toe in sweaters and trousers.

My surgeons had given me the all-clear to sit out in the sun; they were sure the heat would have little adverse effect on my condition, but I was not convinced. As the other children frolicked in the surf on banana boats and pedal boats, yours truly lay prostrate, protected head to toe from the rays.

Subsequent years would see us travel to Majorca again and twice to the Isle of Wight, to the Warner Bros park. I preferred being closer to Old Blighty; the weather was not as hot and I enjoyed the kids' club. Moreover, I cherished the chance to be a normal child again, where nobody judged me by my tumour and I was on a level playing field with Dorothy and Averil. They were happy times and, although it would only be for two weeks, it took us a world away from the trauma of my insomnia back home.

I settled down on holidays, possibly safe in the knowledge that mum and dad were always around me, their days not consumed by work pressures, or worrying about how I was at school or whether I would go down for more than three hours at night.

Frustratingly, though, I can offer no easy explanation why nights were easier on our trips. If I did, I would spend my days writing self-help books to the parents of children with tumours, rather than this meandering autobiography!

Buoyed by the confidence that things were easier on holidays, mum and dad splashed out on more foreign jaunts, treating us to breaks in Portugal, Cyprus and Majorca again in the coming years.

On those trips, my aunt and uncle and their three children joined us, adding to the fun. We have always enjoyed a close relationship with our cousins and the ritual of them coming over from Skye in February to stay with us at Scorrybreck while the parents finalised the plans for the trip in the October half-term break, was almost as enjoyable as the holiday itself.

The foreign trips were testament to Rob's hard work. The long hours, the unsociable house calls at all hours of the day seemed worth it when we were all laughing and fooling around. They were the few times in my life I have felt lucky. And I thank my family for giving me that.

Invariably though, despite the pleasure we took from our family holidays, once home the hostilities resumed.

I was once again sharing a room with Averil. Although separated by three years, in reality I was still the youngest. Free of the problems that beset me, Averil quickly overtook me in physical and educational ability. I sympathise with her greatly now because, although she blossomed into a beautiful sister and is now a wonderful mum, she was deprived the chance to be the baby of the family once I became ill.

While I was in hospital, she was shoved into the background and, once I came home, it was me who took centre stage. Our relationship suffered because of my condition. Before the illness, we were best of friends; inseparable. We had most in common and I cherished the bond we shared, believing it to match the closeness Dorothy and Robina enjoyed. Then, once the tumour took hold, the dynamics of our relationship changed. As I fell behind in school, she progressed. I often felt guilty because her achievements at school, far greater than mine, were constantly overshadowed by the dramas in my life. She soon took the view that she was the older sister.

Today, the added responsibilities she has from being a mother herself have reinforced that view. I cannot blame her.

She has had a lot to contend with and raises her son on her own after the relationship with his father ended before he was born. Even the birth was not smooth. Born without a heartbeat, her little boy's first task on this planet was to fight for his survival. Thankfully, doctors resuscitated him but he was in an incubator for weeks. The fact that he is now thriving is testament to his mother's love and devotion.

I admire her strength now but back then we fought like two ferrets in a sack.

Separated for a while because of my nightly restlessness, we were now back sharing a room. My little sister had no time for my histrionics, believing, like all my siblings that I was only ill when I was in a hospital bed. Any other time, I was fair game. No doubt we would have fought if we were just normal adolescent girls but Averil suspected I played on the tumour and was fed up of mum taking my side in any dispute.

The reason we were back in one room was that we were now running Scorrybreck as a bed and breakfast establishment. Mum had followed her parents' footsteps by taking her first tentative steps into the hospitality trade. She ran it purely as a B&B for one year before, instead, using the rooms to accommodate foreign students working as guides in the local distilleries.

Our summer guests were a welcome addition to the household but they did nothing to improve relations between Averil and I.

In addition, if that were not enough to contend with, it would have taken Kofi Annan to settle differences between Dorothy and me as well. At school, I still tried to cling to her like a limpet, despite her clear annoyance. Where Dot was concerned I could see no wrong. I was blind to her Mickey-taking and deaf to her jibes. Like Averil, she was frustrated at the preferential treatment she perceived I enjoyed at home but it created less of a conflict between us at home.

School, though, was a different story.

Dorothy, not to put too fine a point on it, could do no wrong at Speyside High. Blessed with athleticism and agility, she obviously nicked all the sporty genes from mum and Archie before she was born. She excelled in practically everything she turned her hand to. While I had the get-up-and-go of a sloth, she was Sport Billy – champ at badminton, tennis, running, jumping, skipping, swimming, anything. If there were prizes for breathing, she would clean up. Annoyingly smart to boot, she occupied top spot in most of her classes – a darling of the teachers.

If I sound bitter... that's because I am! Seriously, even without the tumour, I was disadvantaged from the start, trying to follow a star sister like Dot.

To our teachers, she was everything I was not: clever, hardworking, easy going and a good learner. How she managed all that after what she had been through would baffle even the most qualified boffin.

Think about it; her parents split when she's four, she's uprooted to a new town, her big sister is taken from her, she's forced to deal with her little sister having a life-threatening brain tumour and she suffers sleepless nights for six years. By rights, she should be sitting in the corner of a padded room, clutching her knees, rocking to and fro.

Instead, she's now a perfectly adjusted – well, almost – married mother of two delightful kids.

I appreciate everything she has done for me but, while we were at school together, she was impossible to live up to. Unfortunately, I neither had the energy nor the inclination to try emulating her achievements. The four years between us in school might as well have been a hundred we were so far apart. Even when she left school her ghost still haunted me. Teachers were forever telling me how much they wished I had her drive and determination.

Generally, the impact I made with my teachers was on a par with the success I had made with my fellow pupils. I could not get used to the fact they wanted silence in class. To me, work was simply a distraction to the important business of the day – namely yakking and fooling around.

The only subject I showed any aptitude for was English, and I especially relished discussing issue-based texts. Maybe it was because my own illness had made me more aware of the way people could be sidelined by social pressures, I don't know, but it was the only subject to catch my imagination.

Otherwise, generally, I found the academic side of school-work frustrating – it was hard for me to process data. I wanted to do better in class but how could a girl who could not remember if she'd eaten her dinner some five minutes earlier be expected to commit dates of historical battles to memory?

However, in English – where my teacher, Mr Paterson, demonstrated patience of biblical proportions – I remember being taught how to express myself. I was encouraged to talk about my condition and write stories exploring my feelings about my health. In some ways that encouragement lives with me today and can probably be blamed for putting the idea into my head of writing a book.

Still, it helped me put it into perspective. I learned not to be shamed by my tumour and I began enjoying talking about it – so much so, I haven't stopped since then, as my family will testify.

In addition, I found there was no shame in expressing my feelings as and when I experienced them. In my position, I believe life is too short to beat around the bush with pleasantries if they are not warranted. I have first-hand knowledge of how short life can be – too short to waste time. I soon believed that if I wanted to know something I should ask, and if I desired something I would try to get it.

Sadly, some found my directness off-putting. Often I was sure I could see teachers count to ten under their breath when I demanded answers as to why they had marked me so low again. People were unprepared to hear me talk openly about my tumour, or assess my prognosis quite matter-of-fact. It unnerved them. I think many of us are conditioned to believe that people should suffer in silence – they should overcome difficulties in private with quiet dignity and, above all else, they should not impose the stark reality of an illness on to other people, lest they find it awkward.

Well, I am sorry but I do not think that way.

For the most part, I have found people are fascinated by my condition and want to learn more. And, I am more than happy to fill them in.

However, in school, the same frankness caught pupils and teachers alike off guard.

I often found myself in trouble in class because my directness was mistaken for rudeness. Admittedly, sometimes I probably was, but often it is because I do not suffer fools gladly. My approach was unconventional and my teachers could not handle it. They wanted to pigeonhole me and, with Dorothy and Averil excelling academically, demanded answers as to why I was not like them.

Growing up in such a large family, I had to fight to be heard at home. I would do the same in school.

Chapter Eighteen
The Long Road Ahead

In the aftermath of the September 11th terrorist attacks in New York and Washington, Americans flocked to church in great numbers, desperately seeking answers following the terrible atrocities.

It is little wonder people turn to God in times of strife. Ordinary citizens, who in normal circumstances could not be paid to go to church, suddenly turn to the good book in the hope that salvation lies within its pages. If God is sitting at the end of the phone during prayer time, his ear must be bent with all the misery hurled in his direction by people striving for a quick fix. Fewer people these days offer thanks to God on a daily basis. Church pews lie empty as the number of believers dwindles. We blame the Almighty for the world's disasters yet he is the first person we run to when suddenly it us who are in the firing line.

We were no exception.

Mum's faith was tested initially when I first became ill with the hydrocephalus. It pained her heart to see her daughter being put through so much misery. What kind of world was it that allowed children to suffer so much, she thought to herself?

Then, in the children's hospital in Aberdeen, she was faced with sadness that would have brought tears to the eyes of any mother. Looking upon bed after bed, she saw youngsters forced to battle some of the most devastating diseases – leukaemia, cancers and tumours. What world would rob such little ones of their childhood, replacing it instead with trauma usually reserved for adulthood: surgery, chemotherapy and long-term convalescence?

Mum and I probably were too scared to admit to ourselves at the time but each night, before we went to our beds, we turned to the Lord.

I prayed that God would pull me through my operations, prayed for him to look upon this little girl, insignificant in a planet full of people, and show me mercy; cure me of the things that ailed me.

It was what we had always been encouraged to do at school. I even believed that perhaps the reason I was in this pickle was because – while I was giving my pearlies a quick brush and then hopping into bed – my classmates were diligently putting in some overtime with the Almighty to get into his good books. Crikey, I thought; if this is how God treats little girls who forget to say their prayers at night imagine what he must do to the people who took his name in vain or those boys who callously pulled the legs from spiders.

Yet, the more serious the situation became, the less childlike my view of the world became.

Moreover, in the months following the discovery of my second tumour, mum was lost. Stripped of hope, she desperately needed someone or somewhere to reaffirm her faith. Rarely a worshipper in her life, she then looked to the church in a bid for answers to her questions.

Each Sunday, mum and I would visit the local Mortlach Parish Church, where Rob was an elder. I am sure it was a response shared by many people in similar circumstances. If our troubles were the work of a God unhappy with our supposed lack of faith, then we would show obedience. If the health problems bestowed upon me were in some way punishment for our poor attendance then we would learn our lesson, in the faint hope our show of faith would be rewarded. It was a simple trade-off.

Maybe we were guilty of looking for a quick fix. Perhaps we thought that, by showing our faces in church a few times a year, everything would be all right.

In many ways, joining the other parishioners gave us some comfort. The people were always friendly and caring and I am sure I featured in a number of prayers; such was the kindness of local folk. I am grateful for their concern but, on the whole, personally speaking, the experience drained me.

In my simplistic view, because the tumour was still there and because the surgeons had no way to remove it, these were facts showing our prayers were going unanswered.

110

For two years, I turned my back on the church, convinced it held nothing for me. However, with the encouragement of a local parishioner, I returned to bible studies by joining a church youth group, aged fifteen.

Here, I joined a group of people who were very sympathetic to my plight yet, despite being unwavering in their faith, they could not supply me with the answers I needed. Usually we spent the time singing songs, praising God unreservedly without questioning the events that call into doubt his motives or even his existence. I thought, though, that if I attended he would intervene and make the tumour vanish. Sadly, he must have been out to lunch on the days I was there.

To this day, I am still confused about what I believe. I feel there is a God but I don't believe he is a very nice person and not one worth singing to the heavens about every Sunday. I have seen too much sadness and I am still only 24. Putting my own experience aside, my dad's cousin, Averil, who used to cut my hair for my operations died suddenly of a brain hemmorrhage, an uncle lost his fight against cancer, my nephew had to fight for his very existence the minute he was born and my grandpa suffered with poor health for most of my adult life. I think, as a family, we've suffered more than our share of heartache.

Speaking of grief, however, I have to put my hands up and admit that I was responsible for much of the misery at home. I was still inventing new ways to baffle mum.

My forgetfulness was driving her potty. I continued to amaze her by asking for dinner seconds after I cleared my plate. On one occasion, she fed me three full Scottish breakfasts – sausage, egg, bacon, waffles, hash browns – in quick succession. She looked on amazed as I scoffed the lot.

You might ask what a mother was doing feeding her daughter three breakfasts in a row, regardless of how odd I was. However, you have to remember that I was stick thin and the doctors continually feared I was never going to put on weight. So, for mum, she probably welcomed the chance to feed me up, while being slightly alarmed at the circumstances allowing her to do so.

Mum's situation in the town generated a lot of sympathy in Dufftown. During all our travails, the townsfolk were tremendously supportive of our situation and, when it came to fund-raising events for Cancer Research – which mum still organised on a regular basis – they turned out in great numbers. Mostly, the events were great fun but often they were bloody hard work!

One such time was a twenty-mile cycle run around the hills of Dufftown. I managed to rope in Donald Paterson, my English teacher. One of many people I effectively bullied into taking part. For such events I hated people feeling sorry for me or turning up out of sympathy but the more folk I could rope in the better.

Unfortunately, on this occasion, I would regret Mr Paterson's involvement. He was assigned to look after some of my classmates who joined in on the cycle, and me. Since my problems in the saddle I did not hold out much hope of doing well. After only a mile uphill, I was ready to throw in the towel. I am all for raising money for charity but, because of my tumour, I feel out of puff very quickly. I climbed off the bike and announced I could not go another mile. Knowing a Land Rover was not far behind to check on stragglers, it was my intention to hop aboard and meet them all at the finishing line. Sadly for me, Mr Paterson had other ideas. He persuaded me to get back on the bike and carry on. He convinced me to try another mile and then see how I felt. I managed to complete it but that was definitely the limit. Off I got again. My back was killing me, my feet were freezing; the game was up. Still Mr Paterson would not take no for an answer. Back on the saddle I climbed. Only one more mile, he promised. After the third mile, I was ready to drop. Pushed beyond my capabilities, I felt one more turn of the pedals would kill me. I longed for the warm Land Rover so much I was hallucinating, imagining I could see it trundling up the hill behind me.

This was not good enough for my sadistic English sir. With each mile, he coaxed me back onto the bike and twisted my arm to complete another mile. It did not matter that all the way round the hills I moaned constantly and begged for mercy. Every mile, I announced I was never getting back on the bike.

112

Yet, each time, Mr Paterson persuaded me to carry on. Muttering away to myself about how unfair and inconsiderate he was being in making me do it, eventually we got to Dufftown and the finishing line. I could not believe it. I had done it; I had cycled twenty miles on my own. As I collapsed from sheer exhaustion, the smile on my face stretched from ear to ear.

Did I stagger up to Mr Paterson and thank him for believing in me and for pushing beyond my own limitations? Did I hell!

Stubbornly refusing to give him the satisfaction, I was as grumpy as I had been throughout the run, telling mum and my sisters how terrible he had been for making me carry on when I had been ready to collapse. However, inside I was incredibly proud of myself and grateful for Mr Paterson's faith in me. Typically, I think this episode sums me up perfectly. Somehow, despite my fears, I think I have the power of perseverance to overcome adversity but, annoyingly, I am not the type of person to suffer in silence.

Meanwhile my school days were nearing an end. It was little surprise to anyone that I would be leaving at the first opportunity when I was 16. I simply was not built for learning. Although I was not required to repeat a year in secondary school, the gulf between my classmates and me increased every year and, by the time I left, was a yawning chasm.

Leaving school with no qualifications or prospects might have caused other pupils my age sleepless nights, but I suppose I was well ahead of the game in that respect. As far as I was concerned the issue of an education, or lack of it, came a distant second to the state of my health and whether or not I would live long enough to earn a gold watch for loyal service.

My doctors were reluctant to offer a prognosis on how long I had left. Whenever you raise the subject of a brain tumour with strangers, the question on everyone's lips is: "How long have you got?"

Mum always refused to ask. She felt it better not to know. I think, to be honest, the consultants could not give an accurate prediction. They continued to refer me for six-monthly scans, which in turn showed the tumour was growing but at such a slow rate that they were not unduly concerned.

Their advice was always the same. They would defer judgement until the tumour appeared to be causing me distinct neurological problems. To the frustration of mum, Rob and me, they dismissed my panic attacks, sleep problems, headaches, dizzy spells, chronic fatigue and behavioural issues as anxiety, brought on by my failure to adjust properly to the fact I was living with the tumour.

Our meetings with the specialists were scenes from the movie Groundhog Day, where Bill Murray relives the same day over and over again. We would reel off the list of problems still present some six years after my initial tumour operation. Mum would back-up our record of woe with a host of anecdotal evidence to prove we were no closer to solving my problems than we were a day after they discovered the second lesion.

Of course, the consultants conducted themselves profess-ionally but we all got the distinct impression that inwardly they were rolling their eyes, thinking: "Here we go again."

Yet, while they continually strived to offer me medication that might take the edge of my stress, they were never able to provide me with the solution I craved – taking the tumour out. It was all right for them to say that, although the growth was getting bigger, it was not something to worry about. It was not their head, or their tumour. To me, such statements meant only one thing: I was a large step closer to my death. To me, their logic was skewed. They argued that the longer I lived with this in my brain, the better my chances of survival.

I saw it entirely differently. Knowing what had happened to a dear friend of mine whose tumour had grown to the extent it was inoperable, I could still only predict a similar fate. The ticking time bomb in my skull had to go off someday. What if, I thought, the tumour grows so much between scans that by the time the surgeons realise, it is too late?

My moods grew darker and darker. Contrary to the experts' predictions, the longer I lived with the knowledge there was something growing on my brain, the more miserable I was becoming.

Leaving school with no qualifications was of no conse-quence to me, I believed. What was the point in going to college, putting all that work in, only to collapse one day in a lonely student bedsit? What reward would there be in that?

Growing ever more fatalistic, I became obsessed with my own mortality. I was sixteen. Generally, I felt life was slipping away. As my classmates prepared for the exams to propel them into higher education, or took their first tentative steps into the real world with their first jobs upon leaving school, I was in no man's land.

No education, no prospects, no future. I was virtually un-employable, I thought.

The same thoughts must have been going through mum's head because it was she who offered a solution. In the months before I left school, she returned to the retail trade, opening a clothes shop for infants, Babyworld, in Dufftown; primarily with the objective of providing me with full-time employment. It should have been the ideal move; working with my beloved mum in a store, just a few hundred yards from home, guaranteed income and virtually no chance of being fired. Surely it was foolproof? Maybe, but it was not Caroline-proof.

Initially I started going in after school, just before I left, to help mum out and acclimatise myself with the surroundings. It was clear, even then, that this might not be the dream scenario we had both hoped.

I found the work boring and dealing with customers tedious. Whereas mum has always been a natural for the service industry – bubbly, bright, friendly with a caring personality – I was possibly the worst candidate for such a post.

When customers came in with their problems… well, let's just say I was less than sympathetic. If we did not have a particular size in stock my opinion was it was just their tough luck. Mum, in contrast, would dive for the order book promising to have the desired item for them within days.

In addition, I struggled to keep my mind on the job. I could not see the point in hanging around the shop if there were no customers; not when outside in the street it looked far busier. Mum would tear her hair out. One minute she would ask me to keep an eye on the shop floor, while she retrieved stock from the rear. The next she would return to find the store deserted. Confused, she would step out in the street to either find me chatting idly to a passer-by or across in the baker's shooting the breeze with the staff over there.

I was not going to win employee of the month, that's for sure. Plus, if anything, I think I harmed business rather than assisted sales. Never afraid to speak my mind, I would answer bluntly if asked my opinion on baby wear. If I thought a child should never have been seen in a bright green ensemble, I said so, rather than taking the diplomatic view that, as long as the customer is happy, ring it through the till. Mum would gasp in despair as yet another potential customer left the store with their hard-earned cash still intact in their pocket.

Inevitably, seven months after I had left school, it was clear mum's plan to find me work had backfired. Tactfully, mum claimed her heart was no longer in the retail business and she fancied a return to nursing; the profession she had flirted with after leaving school. She was going to sell up Babyworld. I would have to find a job elsewhere. I had no complaints.

However, if I failed to hold down a job with my own mother (who would forgive a multitude of sins) how would I hope to fare with any other employer?

And so, my first job in the real world had ended in spectacular failure. The experience taught me one thing, though; the feeling of rejection that was to become all too familiar in the coming years.

Leaving my mum's employment signalled the start of my roller coaster career ride. My exploits will not put a scratch on the nation's future pension provision but I've done wonders for the economy in the north of Scotland – not least because my sackings always create a new vacancy.

Chapter Nineteen
Wicked Whispers

Knowing mum's shop was closing; I applied for a few local jobs and was delighted when I landed my first interview. I felt like a grown up. It was for a waitress job at one of the biggest local hotels.

The only requirements were being able to hold a large tray of drinks or dinner plates – simple for ordinary people, but enough to fill me with dread. Thankfully, the manager did not want a demonstration before making his decision and I was hired.

At first I revelled in my new role. Although nervous at first, I enjoyed meeting and speaking to guests and took the job very seriously. Being able to assert my personality in a new environment, my clumsiness subsided and I felt quite proficient at delivering drinks and taking orders. The staff was young and friendly and I finally felt I was joining the real world, away from the shelter of my parents or their friends. Sadly though I was to discover the real world can be a nasty place to inhabit sometimes.

Clueless to the intentions of the opposite sex until that point in my life, I had no idea what drove boys or how to play them. With the exception of a few mild kisses, probably the result of a dare on their part, I had managed to make it through school without registering on the radars of any male classmates.

Suddenly, thrown into a situation where people were working long hours together, I was naïve to the subtler points of courtship. After a couple of months, I caught the eye of one of the younger chefs. If he hadn't made the first move, I probably would not have thought twice about him but, once he did, I could not get him out of my head.

I felt flattered and thrilled that a boy was interested in me – and confused too. I was such a stranger to the complexities of relationships that I really didn't stand a chance.

His attempts to woo me stretched as far as sidling up to me one night, after the last drinks were being cleared away and grunting, "You, me. How about it?"

Confronted by such a silver-tongued Lothario as this, how could I resist?

However, once we had agreed we were an item that was when the trouble started. I was only sixteen, and still wet behind the ears. He was seventeen, and painted himself as a man of the world. He probably thought I was a soft touch and looked on me as an easy conquest.

In some ways, he was right. Without a clue what to expect from a relationship, I was just happy a boy knew my name and was prepared to say he liked me. Anything else was a bonus. However, although naïve, I still knew my limits.

It quickly became clear this spotty youth was only after one thing. Skipping the normal rules of courtship, like kissing and holding hands, he cut straight to the chase and demanded we consummate our relationship. This was a dilemma. Unsure of how people normally behaved, I felt pressure to give in but, instinctively, I knew this was a step too far. Confused, I was scared that if I said no, he would dump me, but I was nervous of the consequences if I consented. It's sad to think I was bothered at the time because, obviously, we had nothing between us. I doubt he even knew my surname. Still, I stuck to my guns and held out.

"What's the rush?" I asked. "I barely know you. Why not wait a bit until we're both sure?"

Such reasoning was lost on the brute, who displayed all the evolutionary skills of an amoeba. The more I refused, the more he pestered me. Now, I was scared. Still confused that I was doing the right thing, his aggressiveness unnerved me. Had I committed a cardinal sin? Was this not what young girls were supposed to do? Yet, still, I was not convinced giving in was the solution. Soon, I was to discover my problems were only beginning. What should have been a minor situation between two people suddenly escalated into a full-scale drama.

My "boyfriend" took the rejection personally and, in an act of revenge, started spreading nasty rumours about me around the hotel.

I was gutted. Too inexperienced to know how to react, I wilted. I had no idea about appropriate action I could take. As far as I saw it, he was in with the bricks, even though he had only been there a few months longer than I had.

Conscious of people whispering behind my back, I imagined that every snigger I overheard was aimed at me. Remembering my misery when I had started school, I had been careful to keep word of the tumour under wraps, hoping my new colleagues would accept me for who I was. But once again, I felt like the outsider. Only this time it had nothing to do with my health. As the gossip spread – ironically, lies about my sexual promiscuity – I struggled to retain my composure on duty. I forgot orders, spilled drinks and dropped trays, everything I had tried so hard to overcome.

Eventually, my position became untenable and the manager let me go. I didn't have the heart to speak up. Five months after landing the job, I was back on the scrap heap and yet I was still only sixteen.

The episode depressed me for a while and made me wonder if this was what all relationships were like.

I blamed the tumour for my miserable record with boys. It must give off a scent that repels them, I thought. Certainly, I had been a late developer and my delayed puberty had caused my doctors some concern. At one point they even prescribed oestrogen to speed up my progress. This, I was sure, was the reason I was such an unappealing prospect for the opposite sex. Then, even if they did get past that and started to like me, no doubt the tumour would flare up and cut short love's young dream. Those were the thoughts that kept me awake at night. What man would want to date a woman who could drop dead at any point?

While other girls my age were experimenting with drink and its effect, I rarely socialised outside school and, because I didn't fall about drunk, I took my time to nurture an interest in boys. Instead, I yearned after them from a distance, too scared to declare an interest.

I felt eternally confused – blessed with the emotions that send butterflies to the stomach of every teenage girl, but cursed with the fear of using them.

When I first arrived at high school, I think I desired a different guy each week. During first year I developed an unhealthy obsession with a boy in Dorothy's year and used to follow him around the place like a puppy. Still, maybe that was the first inkling that I would prefer older men!

Like many things when I was growing up, the art of seduction and the mating rituals of men and women seemed all very baffling to me. When my two older sisters brought boys back to the house, I couldn't see the fascination. The girls would tease me about my lack of knowledge regarding sexual terminology. I'd overhear them using words I didn't know the meaning of but I'd try to impress them by repeating them anyway, almost always inappropriately.

Once, Robina brought a boyfriend home to her house in Skye while I was visiting. He stayed overnight and the following morning I wandered into his room. Without so much as a hello or introduction, I politely offered him a very personal service. He sat stunned as I asked again, without the foggiest idea what I would do if he said yes.

Before long though, my health, which had improved in the previous months, once again took centre stage. In August 1998, I was back in Aberdeen Royal Infirmary for my fourth brain operation.

My doctors wanted to replace the shunt I had been living with since I was five. Because I had grown, the coil to my abdomen had stretched and needed lengthening. By now, I treated major surgery in the same way people go to the dentists; it was a necessary evil I had to endure every few years, it seemed.

I recovered well from the operation but, a day after surgery, I began vomiting severely. It was always the drawback of being put under the anaesthetic and I invariably reacted badly to it.

By now, I could recover quite quickly from major surgery and, seeing I was making good progress, my surgeons allowed me to leave just five days after the procedure.

However, I wish I could say that the longer I was living with the tumour, the more settled I became. Sadly, as it had been for the previous few years, the opposite was the truth. I grew more and more anxious.

My consultant neurologist Mr Blaiklock, the excellent surgeon who had removed my earlier tumour in the pineal gland, told me we were entering a "watch and wait game". He would monitor the tumour's progress closely. If he felt it grew to a size that could cause concern then he would take a view to operate. He was clear, though; he would not go in if there were doubts it would do me any good.

It was easy for him to say. It was not his tumour. Although, by then, I was well into my teens, I still viewed my situation with the same childlike innocence I had when I was ten. I just wanted him to remove it. Thinking about what happened to Caroline Nicol – whose tumour was inoperable – still filled me with the dread that I would face a similar fate.

I tried to put it to the back of my mind but it was virtually impossible.

Therefore every six months he would summon mum, Rob and me back through to Aberdeen for my scans.

More often than not, we would not hang around for the results. It always took longer than they predicted. Also, mum grew weary of hearing the same prognosis. Usually they would tell us there was no change, or there was a slight increase in size but not enough for us to worry.

Often, our local GP Dr Heneghan was entrusted with the job of telling us the results.

When I was fifteen, the tumour grew in size in consecutive scans. However, because my neurological signs failed to show any other effect the tumour might be having, they still preferred to hold off.

Over the coming months, we had a number of meetings with Mr Blaiklock. Even though he was a surgeon, and he commanded my utmost respect, I started shouting at him. Why wasn't he doing something? Did he not understand that I wanted it out now? If he left it too long, it might be too late.

In the face of such mad ravings, it was amazing he remained calm. If he went in when there were no indications that I would be better off post-op, he would not risk it. He was confident of spotting the neurological signs that would give him the nod it was time to go in.

121

In all the conversations I had with Mr Blaiklock, although I must have been a precocious little madam, he was always courteous and treated me with respect, talking directly to me as the patient, rather than to mum and dad.

He recognised it was my tumour after all.

He grew concerned about headaches I was experiencing in the early morning and toyed with the idea of bringing me in more frequently for scans. However, he was reluctant; primarily because he knew more scans meant more results, which meant more anxious waiting around. His philosophy was simple. He knew where the tumour was and could roughly gauge how much it would grow.

One subsequent scan picked up abnormalities in my upper brain, around the spot where the growth was. Surely now they would act? No. Once more, because I appeared otherwise healthy, Mr Blaiklock was reluctant to operate – especially if there was a risk surgery could leave me brain damaged.

When I heard this, I went potty. How could he play so fast and loose with my life? Mistakenly, I believed he was acting irresponsibly. Looking back, I sometimes wonder what a teenage girl was doing questioning the reasoning of an eminent brain surgeon, but that's just the way I am. I'll never sit in silence when I think there are answers to be found.

He told me I had to learn to live with the uncertainty. He said the tumour was growing exceptionally slowly and he hoped, in time, I would come to terms with it.

At the time I thought he was nuts to suggest such a thing. I believed there would never be a day when I would accept this situation.

With everything that had been going on – my unhappy work situation, the operation on the shunt and my growing discontent with the tumour – mum decided a change of scene might do me good.

She suggested I go to Skye for a year and live with nana. My grandmother had been on her own since grandpa died two years previously after a long battle with heart disease. She had shown remarkable devotion to her husband, caring for him almost single-handedly in his later years.

I decided to look for work on the island so I would be able to pay my way. It was late winter so I knew many of the local hotels would begin looking for staff, as they reopened for the spring.

The first place I called was the Portree Hotel. After travelling up for an interview, they offered me a job as a waitress. I offered to supply references but, when they heard I was nana's granddaughter, they hired me on the spot. The family name still counted for much on Skye.

Having said that, I don't know what nana was thinking when she agreed to take me in but it was settled. For the first time since I was 18 months old, I was going to Skye to live.

I arrived at nana's full of expectation, hoping the new start would be the tonic I needed to kick start my life.

However, I should have known, given my track record, it could not last. While I was finally getting my life in order, back home in Dufftown, something was about to happen that would rock the family to its core.

I had only been away from home for a few weeks when I was to get the news.

I remember vividly the night when I first suspected all was not well in the Macdonald clan. Nana has two phones, one in the living room and the other in her bedroom. She was talking quietly on the phone in the bedroom one night. By the time she returned to the living room, where I was watching television, it was clear she had been crying.

I looked up at her, hoping my eyes would let her know I was willing to listen. My efforts were in vain. She maintained a mournful silence.

It was not for a full two days later that I found out the reason for nana's reticence. The phone rang. It was dad. Before I even had time to contemplate how unusual it was for him to ring me, he dropped the bombshell.

"Your mum's left home," he said bluntly. "She's with another man."

Chapter Twenty
When Love Breaks Down

His news caught me so off guard, I grabbed for something to stop me keeling over.

"She's what?" I managed to stutter out.

"She's walked out," he repeated. "She's with Gordon."

My brain scrambled. Gordon? Who's Gordon?

In my stunned state I thought he was talking about a neighbour, a man married to one of mum's best friends. That's a strange one, I thought. Then it sunk in. He was talking about Gordon Mackie. The man who had replaced Rob in mum's affections was, ironically, also the man who had taken his job.

I'm sure when Gordon answered the situation vacant advert for an insurance agent in the local paper he could not have predicted the turn his life was about to take. With his own marriage coming to an end, the father-of-two, from Hopeman, believed a career switch to Dufftown might be the life change he was crying out for.

Dad, a workaholic most of his life, was reluctant to give up the job he had successfully built up over twenty years. However, when doctors advised him to take early retirement on medical grounds, he had little option but to go. Rob had been suffering from depression for a while before that and was on medication for stress.

Throughout all our problems, dad had never worked less than twelve hours a day as an insurance clerk. Believing he was doing everything he could to give his family the best possible standard of living, he was exhausted. The trouble was he rarely took a day off. He was always at the disposal of his clients who, as I explained, would not give him a moment's peace. His devotion to the job drove mum mad. She would have given anything for one day a week together.

The tension the situation caused could not be overestimated. One minute they were perfectly civil to each other but the next mum would fly off the handle and claim dad had done something wrong. But he had never done anything wrong. He was a good man, and still is, and would never do anything to hurt his family.

His only flaw was that he was conditioned to work hard. He worked long hours so we got our foreign holiday every year and the best of presents and clothes.

Torn between his duties of providing for his family or freeing up time to spend with his wife, eventually something had to give.

Mum, at first, was delighted. She thought, finally, they would soon be enjoying some overdue time together. It should have been the perfect time for them to rekindle their relationship. However, dad's retirement was not the second summer of love mum hoped it would be. As well as recommending he give up work, his doctor also suggested he take up a hobby, something to take his mind off the stress he was under, completely removed from the day job he'd been doing all these years.

As it was dad took on something that would make even more demands of his time than the insurance job. He reverted back to the life he knew as a child, growing up on a farm. Renting a smallholding, he acquired some cattle and returned to the simple life. The trouble was he was away from the house at the crack of dawn, often not arriving home until after dark. At least with his previous job, he worked from an office in the house. Moreover, if the cows needed tending, there was only one person on call.

As he became more involved with his new project, mum despaired. What good would come out of early retirement if he were to spend all his waking hours at the farm?

It was the catalyst for countless rows. Margaret even accused him of loving his cows more than her.

Initially, the thought of leaving Rob would have been unthinkable. They had been through so much together, not least of all my health nightmares. At one time, she would have followed him to the ends of the earth if they'd just had a day off together once in a while. To her, he was a wonderful father and she worshipped the ground he walked on.

But this was no life. If she had been selfless she would have put aside her desires and stayed with dad for the sake of us kids.

However, she knew she couldn't do that and still remain true to herself. Mum has always believed life is too short not to grasp happiness when you are presented with it.

So, it was little wonder her head was turned when a man came along who would finally show her some attention.

Gordon first came to the house after he'd got the call the job was his. As the job was client based, dad's bosses thought Rob should take in the new start and show him the ropes. Gordon regularly arrived at the house for tuition from dad. He would spend weeks with Rob, learning the system until it was time to take over. He would have been blind not to see the insurance position was not the only vacancy at Scorrybreck.

When mum realised she could not disguise her feelings any longer, she knew it was time to break the news to the family. Being a former nurse, she must have thought that in the same way ripping off a plaster is less painful done quickly, so the short, sharp shock treatment was best. She announced she was leaving to Rob a week before his birthday. The following morning she left Scorrybreck for the last time and headed for her good friend Anne's house nearby.

Averil was next to find out. Coincidently, she was staying over with a friend in the same street. When mum met her she was straight to the point, "I've left your dad. I'm with Gordon now." Averil was speechless. She was in such a state of shock her pal had to ring Dorothy, who was busy working in a local pub. Picking up Averil on the way, she rushed home to find dad in a terrible state. For the second time in nearly twenty years his wife had been taken from him.

By the time he called me, nearly two days later, he was so matter-of-fact. It was as if he was talking about someone else's life; like he was simply imparting an idle piece of gossip.

I was numb. Mum leaving dad. It was unthinkable.

At the time, I had no idea their marriage was in trouble. Yet, looking back, the signs were there. I had just been too obsessed with my own world to see what was happening in front of me. I wondered, when mum recommended I go to Skye, whether she could forecast the upheaval ahead. Perhaps she thought if I was already at nana's and settled into a new life, the split would have less of a devastating effect on me.

As it was, when the break came, I had only been away from home for just over a month.

Questions, obvious to me now, like where was she, what did this mean, were of no concern. Instead, I think I pretty much just said: "Okay then." I don't know whether so much had happened in our family that I was conditioned to switch off at such times; a defence mechanism that had so far seen me able to cope with all of life's stresses. Whatever the reason, I remained calm. I was in a strange situation. Cut off from my sisters, I was alone. Although we often fought like cats and dogs, they were my emotional barometers, useful for knowing what to think and on which side to fall during a crisis. Without them I was left with only my own thoughts. In the immediate aftermath of the phone call, one thing was clear; I couldn't speak to nana about it. I wouldn't dare. She would never hear a bad word about mum.

Perhaps it helped being a bit removed from the situation. I viewed the whole thing philosophically. If my parents were unhappy, I would rather they split than live a lie together. I'm not a great believer in affairs. I realise the course of true love rarely runs smoothly but I think, once you've made your mind up to be with someone, come clean.

Mum moved out and joined Gordon, who split from his wife, in a rented farm not far from Elgin.

The break-up was going to be a test of strength and loyalty for the family. Dorothy, ironically after the stress she'd originally given Rob over Archie all those years ago, became a mountain of support for him during the break-up. Averil, then still only fifteen, was perhaps hit hardest because, for the first time, she was experiencing something the rest of us had been through years previously – our natural parents going their separate ways.

Robina, always very close to mum even though for years they lived many miles apart, had her own life now. When Archie and Shona decided to relocate to Inverness, my eldest sister stayed on at nana's for three years, working in a nursing home. At nineteen, she'd jacked in her job with dreams of travelling to Tenerife to work in a bar with a friend. However, her foreign adventure lasted just a week, when her pal grew homesick and promptly hopped on a flight back to Scotland. Stranded in the tourist Mecca of Playa de las Americas, she called on mum to bail her out and, just two weeks after setting out, returned home. After that, Robina briefly spent some time in Dufftown, while I was still at school, but was itching to kick-start her life. Moving to Elgin, she met the man who would become her husband and, not long after, fell pregnant with her first child. However, their relationship was doomed and even a six-month spell in England failed to save it. They returned to Morayshire once again but, after three years together, decided to call it a day. So, although now she was at least closer to mum, living only minutes away in Elgin, Robina had her own life to worry about and another mouth to feed.

As for Michael, he was always going to side with dad. Much older than the rest of us, he often clashed with mum, even when her marriage to Rob was strong. Michael may have doted on his younger sisters, but it was always clear whose side he would be on regarding mum and dad.

I enjoyed a special relationship with my older brother. Like all little sisters, I looked up to him and thought him cool with great-looking, interesting friends. Once, while I was in hospital, he was distressed to hear unfavourable reports about the canteen food. The following day, as he lived nearby at the time, he cooked me crispy pancakes, put them in a Tupperware dish and brought them into the ward for me. On another occasion, while he served in the Navy, he sent me a get well card, from "your favourite big brother". I laughed, because, of course, he was my only big brother but he always had the knack of making me feel special.

When my parents split, there was never any doubt that I would stand by mum. We had been through so much together. I often asked myself what our family would have been had I not been ill. Would things have been different? The torture I put my parents through – both in hospital and once I was out – must have pushed them to breaking point. That they stood together through the entire trauma says much for them.

It's sad, though, after all they had been through, that it ended like this.

Sadly my decision to show such unquestioning loyalty affected the relationship I had with Michael. He never said as much but I often thought it was some kind of betrayal on my part against dad.

The reality though, was I had little choice. Just as I had depended on mum's support in the past, so it was that I was always going to need it in the future. I had no idea what the tumour had in store for me.

In many ways though, as we entered another difficult phase, I was happy to be out of the firing line in Skye. Here life was in a time warp, free from family squabbles and tension. Even though I was hurting about mum and dad not being together I was determined to make the most of my time up north.

Chapter Twenty-one
The Skye's the Limit

I cannot believe I have come this far in my story without introducing you to my most loyal friend in the world. He has been with me through thick and thin, albeit through different guises. He is more of a spiritual friend, really.

I have mentioned him before briefly without giving him due credit. He is Percy, my trusted teddy bear.

When surgeons first fitted my shunt, Percy was there. When I spent weeks recuperating, Percy was at my bedside. The time I had to have the shunt revised? You get the picture.

He is my comforter in times of strife, my rock. Sadly, he's had to take on many forms. This is primarily because he became a target for those who wished to hurt me – my sisters. Poor Percy became a target for their spite.

My first Percy was a brown bear but I lost him in a café in Aviemore. It was only when we arrived back in Dufftown, I realised someone was missing. I begged mum to repeat the one and a half hour drive back to the skiing capital to retrieve him but, unsurprisingly, she said no. I was four at the time and instead I took a key ring teddy bear to bed, but it was not Percy. Mum and dad, fearful the trauma was going to do me lasting damage, bought me another teddy and I christened him the new Percy. That was the way it worked. If ever I lost him or he was ripped into shreds, the next bear I got would become the next generation.

The Percys took a hell of a beating. Almost without fail they forever needed their arms stitched back on, ears replaced or eye transplants. It didn't help that I took them everywhere I went, slept with them every night and cuddled them relentlessly.

Nana took an instant dislike to Percy III. Coming from a generation that survived the war without the need of security blankets or ragged cuddly toys, she was dismayed at my attachment to this mangy rag. It didn't help that my friend was in a sorry state, his head and arms crudely held on by safety pins. She offered to buy me a new teddy to replace my battered

Percy but I recoiled in horror at the suggestion. One thing was clear from the outset, though, Percy was a marked bear.

Our clash over my beloved toy was an early indication that my stay in Skye was going to be a war of attrition, a battle of wills between nana and me. Used to getting my own way in Dufftown, I quickly learned nana's tolerance for my histrionics was zero. Nana had every sympathy for me but despaired every time mum reported back about my night time terror fits. She always sympathised with her daughter's near impossible situation but, not long after I moved in, I suspected she believed she could knock me into shape.

I was barely in the door when she laid out the ground rules. If I was out I had to be back home at certain times and my meals would be served at set hours every day.

Unhappy at the thought of living in what I viewed as not much more than a prison camp, I originally thought I might be able to move into the hotel where I worked to escape my draconian landlady. However, one look at the dingy room and the dent in my pay packet it was going to make made me return to nana's, where my bed was made, pyjamas were folded and water bottle was always hot. Despite my fears, I grew to love it.

I don't know if it was staying with nana, the fresh sea air, or the fact I was miles away from home but Skye was the tonic I needed. My sleeplessness, although it had subsided since I left school, still caused me problems intermittently. However, in the Hebrides, away from the pressures of my normal life, I relaxed and settled in to a routine quite happily.

I enjoyed working as a waitress in the Portree Hotel and, for the first time in years, started to savour life. I enjoyed the job and because the manager always seemed to be busy, had greater responsibility, answering phones and dealing with guests. I felt I ran the place and never missed a day.

Nana and I continued to have run-ins over Percy, though, particularly when I asked her to stitch his arm on after yet another horror accident. If nana tried to refuse, I threw a tantrum any two-year-old would have been proud of. The tactic usually worked at home but nana was made of sterner stuff. Digging her heels in, she threatened to throw Percy in the bin. Convinced she was merely calling my bluff, I went to work as normal, but when I returned was horrified to learn she'd kept her word. Traumatised, I raked through the bin, trying to retrieve him. Once again, though, nana was one step ahead. Quite smugly, she told me she predicted my reaction and so made a special trip to the Co-op to dispose of him properly.

Not to be outdone, I soon acquired a new teddy. Percy number four. Yet, looking back, the third generation bear made a lucky escape, as his successor took the worst treatment. Dorothy and Robina persecuted the little, white bear. They stapled him to the ceiling, strung him up on a bush and kicked him around the house.

When I was twenty, my boyfriend at the time complained I was too old for a toy. As a compromise I cut his arms off and carried his severed limbs around in my pocket, satisfied that I always had a little bit of Percy with me wherever I was.

This is the Percy who still survives today, but only just.

Anyway, I digress. Percy trauma aside, I was enjoying life on Skye. As spring turned into summer and the nights grew longer, I came to realise what people found so special about island life. I've often thought since then that, if sunshine was guaranteed in our Scottish summer, there wasn't another place on earth I would rather be.

So it was this year. Sometimes I couldn't wait long enough to finish work, head home to nana's for a quick change and a bite to eat, then it was back down into town for a night out.

Life on Skye seemed to be the complete antithesis to what was going on back home. There everyone knew me and those that didn't quickly judged me. However here, no one seemed to bother about my condition. Naturally many people were aware of my background through the family links and the times I'd spent here during the school holidays, but fewer people fussed over me like they did back home.

Mostly, though, I enjoyed my time on Skye because, for the first time, I enjoyed a social life. I tried alcohol for the first time and quickly discovered it did not agree with me.

Having reached the ripe old age of seventeen without a drop of liquor passing my lips, it was inevitable that my first real session would end in tears. As it was, the location for my virgin foray into drunkenness was the Caledonian Hotel – nana and grandpa's first business venture on the island. Trying to negotiate the steep, curving staircase down to the street is a tricky prospect at the best of times, so trying it half-cut was always going to be perilous.

Staggering down the steps, I initially thought I was having a dizzy spell, as the stairs weaved about below me. Three seconds later, I was lying in a crumpled heap at the door, having slid onto my rear and bumped unceremoniously to the bottom. I'd like to think this embarrassing episode at least came after a night of heavy drinking. However, to be honest, I probably only had two Bacardi and Cokes.

The experience did not quite put me off alcohol for life but to this day I have no stomach for a drink, the same measures would have a similar effect on me now.

I'm glad I have never relied on alcohol to have a good time. I enjoy the odd tipple once in a while but, as Dorothy says, I don't need drink. I am like most people are when they've had a skin-full all the time.

I will always cherish fond memories of my time on Skye for other reasons. It was there that I finally had my first proper kiss. It happened in the front room of a boy's house, not far from my nana's. I remember it vividly because Madonna's comeback single 'Frozen' was playing on his television. It was a lovely moment, one I'll savour forever. It didn't lead to anything but it taught me warm feelings could be attached to all this relationship stuff and it didn't have to seem seedy or wrong.

Yet, just as I felt I was finally living the life of a normal teenager, my past caught up with me. Almost without warning, my headaches returned, dull and throbbing like before. Soon, the dizziness followed and, when I went for a hospital check-up, I looked wobbly on my feet. To my astonishment, I failed even the simplest of neurological tests.

The specialists summoned me to Aberdeen again. A scan told them what they needed to know. The tumour had grown.

I was going to need further brain surgery.

Chapter Twenty-two
Every River I Try to Cross

My body's early warning system kicked in as before. The neurological signs my surgeons were looking for started to present themselves during the summer of 1999, shortly after mum and dad split up.

The energy I'd experienced when I first went to Skye was replaced by the tiredness I was all too familiar with. My headaches returned, with the same throbbing menace and my balance wobbled off kilter. Something must have been happening inside my brain, I thought.

My latest scan showed the tumour was now nearly four centimetres, with cysts growing where the surgeons had been before.

Earlier than expected, I was going to leave Skye. The consultant's prognosis was unclear. The operation could take a lot out of me. I could be incapacitated. I might need help with everyday activities like bathing and dressing. Mum immediately said I was to move in with her and Gordon. Such tasks demanded a mother's help. It would be too much to ask Rob to perform such duties.

I returned from Skye and moved in with mum and her new love in their rented farm. Within a week we all moved into a new home in Elgin. For the time being at least, I would say goodbye to Scorrybreck and Dufftown.

On 15th September 1999, doctors readmitted me to Aberdeen Royal Infirmary for operation number five. I was seventeen.

Mr Blaiklock was once again the man entrusted with the job of keeping me alive. He explained it was still too risky to attempt removing the tumour. However, he said, there was an alternative. He could debulk it, meaning he could enter my head and trim a bit off.

The following morning, once again the medical staff prepared me for surgery. He would go in as before, with me sitting up. This method has since gone out of fashion, with some surgeons considering it more dangerous but it was still the favoured option at Aberdeen.

Mr Blaiklock saw two nodules on the tumour. Using a high-tech cavitron ultrasonic aspirator, he bored a hole through the back of my head and began chipping away at the foreign matter. The machine is essentially a fine tube using suction power with a tip that vibrates twenty thousand times a second. As saline flows on the outside, the tiny tube hammers away at the tumour. As the bits are broken away from the main mass, the tube sucks them up. This way, the surgeon removes pieces of the tumour delicately without the risk of harming vital organs. The device was funded by public subscription from generous Aberdonians, who raised double the £80,000 needed for the machine. Its first public demonstration was to Princess Margaret during a visit she made to the hospital. She had looked on amazed as the specialists showed the device sucking yolk from the middle of an egg without touching the white or cracking the shell.

My head was made of slightly thicker stuff, but Mr Blaiklock achieved results with just as much ease and precision. His problem was knowing when to stop. If he went too far, he could enter the brain stem and cause irreparable damage. Once satisfied he had safely removed enough of the tumour, he halted the procedure. Tests on the matter recovered from my brain confirmed it was a cystic fibrillary astrocytoma – a tumour comprised of fibres and composed of supporting cells commonly seen in children. Now, at least, I knew my enemy.

After the op, I recovered consciousness quickly enough but took a while longer to regain my full senses. As usual, I felt ropey coming out of the anaesthetic. I recovered in Ward Forty in the main hospital; a stark reminder I was not a child anymore. The realisation then hit me that this condition was going to follow me into adulthood.

As I recuperated in my bed, a woman in the same ward caught my eye. She was another patient, from Stornoway, on the Isle of Lewis. She was in a terrible state, tossing and turning and ranting away in Gaelic in her bed. I did not know the woman but she seemed distressed and could not settle. I offered her my portable CD player. I had been listening to my Runrig albums, featuring their former lead singer Donnie Munro, a fellow resident of Skye, who lived just down the hill from nana. Immediately, the Gaelic voices on the CD and the lilting melodies soothed the woman and calmed her down. She was extremely grateful and wanted to know all about the band - whose music had settled her.

Runrig, at the time, were one of Scotland's top rock acts, their blend of heartfelt Gaelic/English tunes winning them an army of fans across the globe. I had always taken an interest in them, but especially so after my uncle introduced me to Donnie. I'll always remember that day. I had a book on the band, which my uncle suggested we take down to Donnie's for him to sign. He invited us into his house, which boasted stunning views of the bay across to the Cuillin Mountains rising in the distance, and led us through to his dining room where he has a grand piano. To my amazement, Donnie treated me to a rendition of my favourite Runrig song "Every River". With typical brass neck, I asked him if I could perhaps sing live with him sometime. Fully expecting a polite refusal, I was further stunned when he said, "Sure, why not?"

Donnie was true to his word and arranged for me to join him for the sound check at one of his future shows. The concert he had in mind was no ordinary gig – it was his final appearance with the band at Stirling Castle in 1997.

On the day of the show, I had butterflies in my stomach as I travelled down with mum and some friends. We picked up our VIP passes at the gate and met Donnie just as he was about to commence their final rehearsal for the big night.

Standing on stage next to my hero, I got such a rush. Although we were only playing to a select audience of roadies and technicians, when Donnie handed me the microphone it felt like I was a real pop star, playing in front of 50,000 adoring fans.

We sang "Every River" once more. I was a bag of nerves and probably sounded awful. My only other experience of singing live in public was at one of mum's Cancer Research fund-raisers, when I let rip with a decidedly ropey "Anything You Can Do, I Can Do Better".

When Donnie and I finished our duet, the assembled party clapped appreciatively, probably relieved it was over. Our VIP treatment did not end there, however. Donnie had arranged for us to watch the gig from the side of the stage, looking out on to the throng. It was wonderful to play such a prominent part in a historical moment in the band's career and I'm indebted to Donnie's kindness. Since then, he's only ever been a phone call away from me and, despite his busy lifestyle, always seems happy to talk to me.

Demonstrating that thoughtfulness, he called me up in hospital after the debulking operation. The switchboard put him straight through to Ward Forty, where a nurse transferred him through to the phone by my bed.

It was wonderful to hear from him and I was touched not only that he remembered I was in hospital but that he was taking time out to check how I was. Before he rung off, I passed him to the woman who had loved his music the previous day. I simply told her someone was on the phone who would like to speak to her. The two of them chatted away and she came off saying what a nice man he was. She asked who the delightful young chap was but was gob-smacked when I revealed Donnie's identity.

Following surgery, my consultant's prognosis offered me some small comfort. The tumour, although still there, was greatly reduced in size. Essentially, however, we were still in the "watch and wait game". So again, for the foreseeable future, my life would consist of regular scans and close monitoring. The consequences of following any other course of action would be fatal.

Despite my surgeon's fear before surgery that the procedure might leave me incapacitated for some time, I defied their predictions and made a speedy recovery. The specialists wanted to keep me in for observation but the steady stream of visitors to my bedside helped pass the hours and days.

Among them was Archie, who popped in to see how I was doing. Dear old 'real dad', as I like to call him, always kept abreast of my progress – mostly via Robina and nana.

It was tricky for him. Practically persona non grata in mum's eyes, he probably suspected he should keep a wide berth when it came to issues around me. My adoption pushed him further to the background and he recognised Rob's place in my life.

However, with mum splitting from Rob, he possibly felt it a bit easier to play a more visible role. Recently separated from Shona, he was living in Inverness, closer to hand and with more time to devote to visiting his somewhat estranged daughter.

I was delighted to see him, as I was with all my visitors. It takes an extended stay in a hospital bed to appreciate the family you have – and I have more than most. Of course, mum was still an almost constant presence by my bedside, and would often make the trip over from Elgin with Gordon. Dad would also journey from Dufftown, sometimes with Anne, mum's old friend. Margaret and Anne had been bosom buddies since early adulthood and Anne had played a pivotal role in the early days of my illness, offering valuable support to mum when she was most up against it.

It was during such a trip to see me that Anne became reacquainted with Archie. They bumped into each other during visiting hours and – besides feeling concern for yours truly, of course – made arrangements to meet up. Goodness knows what mum thought of their relationship when they first started dating – her best friend and her ex-husband getting together. She probably had to bite her tongue on a number of occasions but perhaps, following on from her own change in circumstances, was more inclined to live and let live, rather than dredge up previous heartache. That's one thing I give mum credit for; regardless of her own opinions about people, she does not let her own experiences pollute another's judgement. She would rather folk make their minds up instead of being influenced by her.

Within a few weeks, the surgeons gave me the all-clear to return home. It was strange leaving hospital and not making the journey to Dufftown as we'd done so many times in the past. However, Gordon did everything to make my welcome home as pleasant as possible, carrying me up the stairs to my bedroom after we had pulled up at the house.

Yet another episode in what seemed like a never-ending story of operations and hospital visits was over. Hopefully my tumour's ability to strike me down had been neutered for now. How long it would be before it grew to its former size was anyone's guess. I couldn't allow myself to live forever wondering "what if". Staying with mum and her new partner in a new house signalled the latest chapter in my life. It was about time I started living.

Chapter Twenty-three
Stupid Cupid

The first thing on the agenda was finding a man. The few brief flirtations I had enjoyed on Skye only whetted my appetite for more of the same.

I was eighteen, rejuvenated after my recent health scare and, once again, I felt I had yet another chance at life. If I had been born a cat, I would have been on my fifth life by now. I would not leave it until my ninth to start enjoying myself.

My sleep problems now a distant memory, I felt confident in my new surroundings and I pushed the fear I once held that my condition could only mean heartache for a prospective boyfriend to the back of my mind.

Next on my list of priorities was a job. Buoyed by my recent experiences in the hotel, I felt confident I could land a job I enjoyed and keep it. Sadly, the reality would be somewhat different and my forays into full-time employment would be the first steps on a career path built on quicksand.

Believing my calling was to be a waitress, I secured a post in a café right in the heart of my town's main shopping centre. Thinking its location not only put me at the heart of the bustling retail community but was also a prime position to eye up the local talent, I seized the opportunity. Crucially, I had not paid enough attention to the dress code when I applied for the position. My enthusiasm lasted all of five minutes and, once my boss handed me the regulation straw hat, I realised I would look as appealing to Morayshire's young bucks as an Amish milkmaid. Struggling to conceal my embarrassment, I could never master the job while constantly cringing at my attire. After only four weeks, I'd had enough. Gordon kindly informed them I had decided to pursue my career elsewhere.

Trading the service industry for manufacturing, my next role was on the production line at the local biscuit factory. The company's famous tartan tins are as synonymous with Scotland as dreary weather and tightly tied purse strings. My crucial role in the chain was to put the freshly packaged shortbread into bigger boxes. It was not exactly the most taxing job in the world but, to me, it may well have been quantum physics. The boxes hurtled towards me from the conveyer belt at such a rate of knots that no sooner had I packaged one than hundreds more piled on top of me. As my bosses lectured me on the concept of bottlenecks, they ordered me, in no uncertain terms, to speed up. Yet the more I tried to rush, the slower I became. I lasted all of one day; the boss deciding my job was worth less than meeting the day's production targets.

Next up was a job in one of the world's biggest fast food companies, making burgers that vaguely resembled the picture on the board and shoving them into brown bags. For two months, I settled in well, got along with my colleagues and enjoyed the work. Then, on a night out, disaster struck. I became hopelessly drunk and my boss, although married and much older, took a shine to me. Before I knew it, we were getting it on in his car. Shamefaced, I returned to work anxious about how my indiscretion would affect my job. Initially, it seemed the perfect career move. My boss moved me onto the somewhat cushy drive-in window, even turning a blind eye when my long conversations with dishy customers caused queues beyond the car park.

Soon though, word of our transgression leaked out and spread like wildfire round the restaurant. Typically, although the one seduced, I bore the brunt of the gossips' wrath. Stickers started appearing on my locker, calling me a "dirty slapper". The wickedness upset me. I couldn't understand why I was the target for the abuse. Once again, I was finding out the hard way that dalliances with colleagues could bite you on the backside. Clueless to workers' rights, I let the bullying get to me and decided to leave rather than face the sneering comments any longer. I knew nothing of grievance procedures, tribunals or the options available to me to take action against my boss or the people who persecuted me. Miserable and hurt, I quit, only three months into a job I liked.

Previously I would have retreated into my shell and felt sorry for myself. However, I dusted myself down and, walking out of the firm for the last time, promptly strode across the road to their bitter rival and secured a job there that day. I was to start in less than a week.

Delighted that I'd managed to resolve an unhappy situation all by myself, I endeavoured to tackle the other great quandary in life – how to get a bloke.

It seemed clear I had two options: sit around and wait for Mr Right to come and find me; or get out there and seek him out myself.

To celebrate my freedom from my horrible employers, I hit the town's pubs with some friends, full of expectation. Drinking in a bar called Downtown I spied a potential candidate at the bar. Standing at over six foot, he looked air force material; the local base at Lossiemouth providing employment for hundreds of RAF men.

To the delight of my pals, I commandeered the next round and strode purposefully to the bar. My prey locked in my sights, I brushed aside my fellow drinkers, carefully manoeuvring myself into a position to strike. For a few moments, I waited, full of expectation that, now I was so close beside him, it was only a matter of time before Cupid's arrow struck.

The seconds ticked by. Normally, having the stature of R2-D2, I wait for hours at bars to be served. Typically, that night, when I was looking for an excuse to linger, the barmaid fast-tracked me to the front of the queue. I scowled. I bet the hussy smelled my desire and, keen to land this alpha male for herself, would try anything to kill off the competition.

I looked up at him – definitely future husband material. Still, there was no flicker of lust in his eyes. Stalling, I threw a curveball order at the barmaid, hoping my request for Mexican Goat Juice liqueur would have her scouring the shelves for days. That would buy me time to come up with a line, I thought. Amazingly, she was back in a flash.

"Slice of lime with that?" She smiled triumphantly, meanwhile flicking "shag me" eyes at my man.

Of course, that's when he responded – cocking an eyebrow in appreciation of her bar keeping dexterity.

Crikey, I was up against Aphrodite herself.

Realising I was in the match of my life, I decided it was time to take matters into my own hands. Knowing I would only have one shot at glory, I had to come up with the mother of all chat-up lines, a killer move that would both capture his attention and render him powerless to resist my charms. God, if he was listening, would have to bless me with the very words Adam used to charm Eve. Finally, it came.

"Goodness, you're tall."

That was it. That was the best I could come up with. Looking down, he flashed me the look a cow gives a fly shortly before flicking it from his back with his tail.

"Bet you'd be first pick in any basketball team," I ventured, shutting my eyes, preparing for the inevitable put down. None came. Instead, the only sound greeting my ears was laughter.

"You're cute. Can I get you a drink?"

It had worked. I was in! Gratefully taking him up on his offer, I faced the barmaid, now wearing the look of defeat.

"Ha, ha," I thought. "I am the lioness of love. Hear me roar!"

My new mate, Stuart, was indeed in the RAF; an electrician who tinkered with planes no less. Six years older than me, he seemed worldly and wise, a man, as opposed to the boys I had only experienced before then. We hit it off that night and arranged to meet during the following week. My heart soaring, I floated home that night. Cupid had finally hit the mark.

Before our first date came along, I started my new job. Maybe it was the angels playing with my heart, I don't know, but I got off to a great start in my new workplace. Although it was quieter, it suited me fine, my workmates were friendly and I settled quickly.

Meanwhile, things were going equally well with Stuart. We found our routine, going for drinks, nights out at the pictures, all the things I heard normal couples did.

Sadly, although blissfully happy with my private life, the same could not be said for work. My career curse struck again shortly after my boss moved me to the drive-through window. The headset they made me wear hurt my ear. Despite explaining my health history, my boss ordered me to carry on. Every time a customer bellowed an order, their voice reverberated round my brain. The more I pleaded with the manager to spare me the pain, the more he dug his heels in. Even when my ear became infected and my doctor prescribed medication, he would not listen. Although this was only a few years ago, society was not the disciplinary driven culture it is today and, once again, I had no idea I could report my boss for cruelty. Frustrated that my complaints were falling on deaf ears, I quit. I had lasted only two months.

Still, this latest setback was not enough to keep the new me down. When you're enjoying the love of a good man, which I thought I was, it was impossible to be disheartened about anything for too long.

For the first time in my life, I thought I knew what love was, and it was great. On the arm of my six-foot four-inch RAF man, I felt indestructible, which, given my recent history, was an unbelievable feeling. He treated me the way I thought women should be, taking me to restaurants and hotels. I didn't know it then but he did have an ulterior motive for booking overnight rooms. RAF rules forbid him to take a woman on base and I would never have dared take him home to mum's. She did not say as much, but I was not brave enough to test her resolve when it came to bringing lovers home. I don't know whether I subconsciously wanted to be closer to him but something prompted me to seek a job on his base and, after just nine days out of work, I became a cleaner at Lossiemouth.

On the face of it, manual labour might have sounded like hard work but the reality was it proved to be one of the easiest jobs I had tried. Responsible for cleaning the living blocks, I probably only had a mop in my hands for five minutes in any hour. Always one easily distracted, invariably I would strike up a conversation with whoever was on night duty. Once I coaxed them into making me a cup of tea, I'd put the mop to one side and engage in idle chit-chat.

Another advantage was that I could steal some forbidden moments with Stuart. It was exciting to be smuggled into his living quarters like some illicit lover. An added bonus was that it then only took me five minutes to be at my post in the morning. The trouble was, even with sleeping on base, I still endeavoured to turn up forty-five minutes late.

Inevitably, this led to run-ins with my boss who despaired at my tardiness. She could also see through my pathetic attempts at cleanliness and my inspections always resulted in a severe dressing down.

It was only a part-time job so, to earn more money, I took another position for a few hours in a restaurant in Elgin. It was one of those chains of themed diners, which were popular in the early nineties but suffered a popularity dip once people realised battered old Coke signs and train sets above the bar were not necessarily indicators of class.

As you will no doubt expect, I won no awards for loyal service. I think I only lasted a month. Never known for my diplomacy, I answered the only way I could when a couple of customers asked if I'd recommend the soup.

"Well, I had it for my lunch and it was crap," I said, unaware the manageress was standing right behind me. She gave me the time it took to get my coat to leave the restaurant.

It is just as well I have conditioned myself to accept rejection graciously, otherwise I'd be locked up by now. By the time I received my marching orders from my latest occupation – my ninth in two years – I began to assume jobs were simply short-term projects to keep people off the streets. It didn't matter to me. I was happy at home, having adjusted to life with mum and Gordon far more easily than I had expected.

My relationship with Stuart was also going well, as far as I knew anyway.

Still clinging to my post at Lossiemouth and dividing my time between Elgin and my lover's lodgings, I felt at last I'd cracked this life game.

I should have known that the moment I feel settled with my lot, that's the time something comes along to flip my world on its head.

Sure enough, I did not have long to wait for the next bombshell. I probably should have guessed, but it was mum who again caught us all by surprise.

Since moving to Elgin, she had returned to her first career, working in a local nursing home. Yet, despite the satisfaction she felt of earning for herself, she was disillusioned with the long hours and little reward. Gordon, meanwhile, was out of work after giving up the insurance job – the perfect circumstances for a life change. One night she sat me down and explained that I would soon need to find somewhere else to live.

She was starting a new life; in Spain. She and Gordon would be leaving in April.

Chapter Twenty-four
Staring into the Abyss

Mum's decision to leave Scotland shocked me almost as much as her split from dad. She made no secret of the fact she preferred the warmer climate of the continent and holidayed frequently in the south of Spain.

It was during one such break that she and Gordon met an English businessman who made his living running caravan parks for British ex-pats. He wanted mum and Gordon to run one of these parks, near Benidorm.

Her decision might have stunned me but, for mum, it was an easy one to make. Gordon and she were in a transition zone, each of them having recently left the lives they had known for nearly twenty years. What difference did it make if they were in Spain or Skye. With the advent of low-cost airlines and direct flights from Scotland, it was almost as easy to get to southern Europe as it was to reach the Western Isles.

The elements in mum's life that would normally have tied her to her native country were dissipating by the day. She saw me settled in a relationship, with a job. She believed my dependence on her was the lowest it had ever been.

We would all be able to visit and, when we came to Spain, we would have a base from which to explore the country. It would be an opportunity for us all. Certainly mum had no problem talking up the move. It did not make it any easier for me to take though.

The thought of mum leaving scared me to death. I felt she was abandoning me, finally throwing in the towel after all I'd put her through.

I couldn't deny that, technically, I was in a stronger position than I had been for years, but if my experience had taught me one thing, it was that, whenever I felt most secure, that was when I was most vulnerable.

Neither of us could know what was round the corner.

I also had the added complication of finding somewhere to live. Restricted from moving in with Stuart full-time, unless we were married, I faced living on my own for the first time. After scouring the "to let" ads in local newspapers, I found a room in a flat in Lossiemouth, sharing with a man and his girlfriend.

Shortly before they were due to leave, mum and Gordon, having sold the house, moved in with Robina, who was living as a single mum in Elgin. Mum organised a leaving party in a local function hall called the Cat's Whiskers, primarily for the people she was leaving behind at the nursing home, but also attended by Robina, Dorothy, Averil and me. It was billed as a big celebration, but I did not want to pop champagne corks. As everyone around me laughed and danced, I sat miserable. When I looked at mum smiling, I thought it must be relief; she was finally ridding her life of her problem child, cutting the albatross from round her neck.

On the day before they finally departed, I went up to Robina's house to wish her good luck. Even though that was it, she was leaving Scotland for good, it was a strangely un-emotional parting. Stifling the torment inside, I wished her well. With that, I left her to make the final preparations for her trip. There did not seem any time nor need for sentiment.

In the days following mum's departure, I sunk deeper into depression. Alone in my cramped room, I was cut off from all my family, each of them busy getting on with their lives. Stuart, who had no time for my moods, gave me a wide berth rather than attempting to lift my spirits.

Lying awake at night, I replayed my life like an old cine movie, the images from my childhood flickering across my mind.

There was the school sports day, the trips to the doctor, mum shouting to be heard that something was seriously wrong with me. Then, my operations, waking up to see her, the tenth birthday party and the joy on her face that I'd made it to such a landmark date. Even through the hell of the aftermath, when I drove everyone mad with my panic attacks at night, she stood by me, sympathising with my inner torment. After my latest operation, it was mum who stepped in to look after me, ready to care for me around the clock if necessary. I didn't know at the time that was as far as it went. I did not know a mother's love was only a finite resource.

It appeared everyone had finally had their fill of me.

As the movie in my head flickered to an end, what else was I to do? Clutching a bottle of paracetamol, I poured a glass of water and, methodically, popped each one into my mouth and gulped them down. In my confused, depressed state, there seemed no alternative. At least this way, I was going out on my terms. The tumour would not have the final say in my destiny. The last pill swallowed, I slumped on the sofa, waiting for the darkness to descend. Whatever the afterlife had in store for me, it had to be better than the hand I'd been dealt with in this life. I closed my eyes, wondering if there would be a sign the pills were working, or whether I would simply succumb to the eternal night.

When the phone rang I jumped out of my skin. It was a split decision; stick or twist? Do I answer and cry for help, or let it ring off and await my fate? I chose the former. It was Stuart.

"What are you up to?"

"Not a lot. Just taken a bottle of paracetamol."

"You've what?"

"I've taken a bottle of paracetamol."

"You serious? What did you do that for?"

"Can't go on. Had enough. I hate my life."

"Are you being serious? How many did you take?

"Dunno. I finished the bottle."

"This better not be a wind-up. Christ, I can't leave you alone for five minutes! I'll be right over."

Hmm, not exactly the sympathy I was hoping for.

By the time my one-man cavalry arrived, the nausea was kicking in. So much for praying for a peaceful passage to the other side – I'd be on my knees, certainly, but most likely hurling down a toilet.

Stuart drove me to Dr Gray's Hospital. I could see the embarrassment on his face when he explained to the receptionist what was wrong. If I received little sympathy from my boyfriend, I got even less from the staff.

Two hours later, feeling decidedly ropey, a hospital shrink gave me a dressing down, saying how stupid I was.

She was right, of course. My attempt at suicide was pathetic, a shameful attempt to shock my family. What did I want? Them to give up any chance they have of a life to be at my disposal?

Confiding in Robina, I apologised and hoped news of the incident would not filter back to mum in Spain. If that happened, I would be better off dead.

It was not long before I got the call.

Mum tore through me like a dose of salts, and deservedly so. After all she had done for me, it was a despicable attempt at a guilt trip.

One thing the episode taught me, however, was that I had to get out of my miserable living arrangement.

The solution was to move in with Robina. With the exception of a few months, when my big sister moved in to Dufftown, following her disastrous flit to Tenerife, this was the first time I had spent any prolonged time with her. Thankfully, I am quite a tidy person, who takes pride in her surroundings. I wasn't always like that, however. When Robina arrived in Scorrybreck, her sisters' laziness stunned her. Not having the luxury of a dishwasher at the time, we simply piled our dirty plates in the sink, expecting someone else to clean them. Robina, though, promptly picked them up and dumped the offending crockery in each of our bedrooms.

Mindful of her strict tidy policy, I was on my best behaviour. It was fun living with Robina. We lived our separate lives mostly but I enjoyed hanging out with her and her son, Kyle. I paid her rent, when I was able to, and rented out a single room in her house. She was more accommodating when it came to letting boyfriends stay over so my visits to Stuart on the RAF base tapered off.

Unsurprisingly, the shoddiness of my work at the base became an irritation too far for my boss who summarily dismissed me. In truth, it amazed me that I'd lasted so long. I was back on the scrap heap after my almost obligatory three months.

I added cleaning to the list of jobs it seemed I was not cut out for. I tried to take more care next time round, thinking about a job I would like to do, rather than one out of necessity. A filling station, near to Robina's house, looked like fun. To most people, working in a petrol station might seem a drudge, ringing through sales in rapid fire, while watching for fuel dodgers. Yet to me it appeared the ideal opportunity to speak to lots of different people and, at the same time, take a nosey at what people bought.

When it came to completing the application form, I did my usual and ticked the box indicating I had no medical issues. Just wanting to be normal, I did not want to give prospective employers a reason not to hire me. It never ceased to amaze me when I got the call to say the job was mine, and this time was no exception. I started immediately. The station's location meant it was not a hassle to get to, even for the unpopular night-time shifts, starting at 10pm, or the early shift, beginning at 7am. Sure enough, I started to enjoy it. I love people watching, guessing the stories behind their actions. I would wonder who the man in the expensive suit was buying flowers for late at night – his wife or mistress? When a slightly dishevelled man came in picking up a bottle of wine on his way home, I imagined the stress he must be under to drink alone in the evening.

Sadly, my intention of keeping my tumour from the manager backfired. I was working at the filling station shortly before my shunt blocked, and I needed emergency surgery. In the weeks leading up to it, I started suffering splitting headaches, impossible to mask at work. As my manager raised questions about my health, someone helpfully put him in the picture about the tumour. Rather than making an attempt to understand my situation, he summoned me into his office.

"I'm afraid things aren't working out," he said. "I'm going to have to let you go."

Naturally, he could not say he was firing me because of the brain tumour, therefore leaving himself wide open for a discrimination claim, but I knew the reason. Ironically, this was one job where I always turned up on time, handled the demands of the job and was perfectly polite to customers. Weeks later, while I was in hospital recovering from the shunt blockage, my suspicions were confirmed when Robina popped in to pick up my final pay-cheque. As she walked in she heard the staff discussing my surgery in great detail.

I was wrong to cover up such a serious health condition but that episode illustrated exactly the prejudice I was up against.

My emergency op was to cost me another job. On the day the shunt blocked, I was due to start at a local Indian restaurant. When I failed to show for my first shift, the boss fired me – just another to add to the list.

In the aftermath of my emergency surgery, I was furious that doctors failed to spot the telltale signs that my shunt had blocked. Enraged, I instigated legal proceedings against the out-of-hours service whose negligence I felt nearly cost me my life. Defending their position, Moray Docs, who provide the emergency medical cover, claimed that, while nurses failed to treat my situation with the seriousness it deserved, the doctor did everything in his power to assist me.

Unsatisfied, I notified newspapers of the incident and was amazed when national papers like The Sun and Daily Record took on my case. This was the first inkling that my condition held an interest far beyond the confines of my family.

At school, I had been encouraged to talk and write about my tumour, to express myself and not to be afraid to discuss the implications of my health problems. Since then, I've written about my life in several magazines. It always surprises me when the media take an interest in my plight but I am grateful for their support.

As I was to find out, the wheels of justice turn slowly, if at all. There would be no quick resolution to my battle for compensation, despite the interest from national press. I was forced to give up the fight because my application for legal aid was refused.

Chapter Twenty-five
Homeward Bound

Just as every girl dreams of a fairytale wedding, with a gorgeous white dress and a handsome groom, so they also wish their father is there to give them away, with their mother weeping close by.

Dorothy was no different. Although she knew, when she announced her nuptials to long-term love Harry Officer, that her parents were living separate lives, she prayed they would set aside their differences for her on her special day.

She wanted her natural father to be there, of course, but was also keen to show due respect to the man who had raised her, Rob. The thought of having mum and him in the same room together, however, filled her with trepidation. To give my parents their due, they were all on speaking terms with each other and accepted each person's right to be there. However, with our family, one thing we guarantee is that nothing is simple.

As Rob helped contribute to the costs, it was expected that many of his friends from Dufftown would attend the wedding in Elgin on 1st September 2001. Such friends were loyal to the last and, disapproving of the way mum treated Rob, made it clear her presence was not welcome.

Dorothy was in a tricky situation. Desperately wanting her mum to see her wedding day, she was also careful not to upset the man who had raised her from the age of four.

In the end it was left to mum to make the ultimate sacrifice. From her new home in Altea, southern Spain, she called Dorothy and made the decision for her. She would not attend the wedding. That way, Rob's friends could attend, safe in the knowledge they would be spared an awkward reunion with mum, and Rob would save face on this important day.

While gutted at the compromise, Dorothy could see mum's logic.

And so, while her daughter added the finishing touches to her dress and prepared to take her vows in Elgin registry office, mum was sitting on the beach alone with her thoughts. For the duration of the ceremony and reception, she sat watching the waves ebb and flow, hoping they carried her thoughts back to Dorothy in Scotland.

The wedding passed without a hitch. My sister looked blissfully happy as she committed herself to Harry. I'd always had a soft spot for her groom, even though I did my best to kill off their blossoming relationship while it was still in its infancy. On my first meeting with firefighter Harry at Scorrybreck, in my usual inimitable style, I gave him the once over before laying into his dress sense. Seizing upon the seventeen-year age gap between them, I tactfully said, "Aren't you old enough to be her granddad?" Poor Harry went home that night and immediately binned the trainers and shirt that caused me such offence.

It's a wonder they sent me an invite at all.

Although still with Stuart, I attended alone. He deemed England's crucial World Cup qualifier was a more important game than the love match being conducted down the road from the pub.

It was not the first – and certainly not the last – time I questioned his commitment to our relationship. Although Stuart was quick to act when I downed the painkillers and helped when the shunt blocked, there were many times when he was posted missing.

Blind to it at the time, I now see he was happy to use me. I was convenient for him, always available at the drop of a hat, whereas he, on the other hand, frequently cried off for seemingly trivial matters.

The simple fact was it was a relationship in name only. From the early days, when I accompanied him to RAF Christmas parties, we had since downgraded to sex buddies. If I was honest with myself, it had been a long time since I could truthfully have labelled him my boyfriend.

I should have turned and fled after a bizarre incident when he invited me down to his home in the Midlands. When I arrived, he announced he was having a barbeque in the garden with some friends. He led me upstairs, and showed me to an attic room. "Stay here," he said. "I'll come up and check on you. There are books, magazines and a TV to keep you occupied."

For the duration of the afternoon, I sat abandoned in an attic, while I could hear him laugh and joke with his friends down below. He even locked me in the room so I would not join him and cramp his style.

It sounds ridiculous when I retell it that I tolerated such terrible behaviour but I had no frame of reference for comparison. Stuart was older and convinced me he was wise in the ways of the world. Well travelled and educated, I believed that what he said went. Despite his obnoxiousness, he made me feel safe and secure and, for the most part, wanted; powerful emotions to invoke in a naïve nineteen-year-old girl.

So desperate was I to be loved, I mistook his passing interest as the real thing. Blind to his failings, I only saw or heard what I wanted to fit my dream of how our relationship should be.

It was to get worse.

Around Christmas time, three months after Dorothy's wedding, I dutifully spent days selecting appropriate gifts, lovingly wrapped each one individually, in preparation of our exchange ceremony. However, when I presented them to him, Stuart coldly rejected them. He said he did not want to bother with gifts this year. Without questioning his reaction, I had no option but to return the items to the shops. Then, in a moment that shames me still, I even bought my own Christmas card and signed it from him, knowing there was no chance I'd receive the genuine article.

Despite even that humiliation, we still soldiered on. Stuart joined me when I travelled to mum's the following Easter.

Then, when I took a child-minding job, which required me to move full-time into a remote house in Kellas, several miles from Elgin, I asked him to join me. I should have known, when he turned up with the tiniest of rucksacks, containing only essentials for a couple of nights, that he was not in it for the long haul. But, when he was lying in my arms, I kidded myself everything was all right, that we were like every other couple. I believed this was how adult relationships should be.

It didn't occur to me to worry when he would lie about what he'd been up to. If I mentioned that Robina had spotted him out in a pub, he would strenuously deny it, accusing my sister of mischief making.

We were both too weak to end it. I probably would still be with him today if he hadn't finally taken steps to finish it. Still, though, he wasn't man enough to do it right.

First, he changed his mobile phone but refused to give me his new number. Rather than take the hint, I was determined to prove it would take more than that to get rid of me. Knowing his car was being serviced in the local Volkswagen dealership, I called in at the garage saying I needed something from my boyfriend's car. The unsuspecting staff gave me the keys and, when I then said I couldn't find what I was after but could they give me his number, they duly handed over the elusive mobile digits. Furious I had gone behind his back, he then said the RAF planned to transfer him to Odiham, in Hampshire. He had lied. When I rang the base looking for him, the switchboard operator informed me he was actually in Northern Ireland.

Finally, it hit home. He did not want me to speak to him. After nearly two years, it was over. I was besotted with him. I thought I loved him but it was clear he didn't love me. Now, thankfully, I know what love is, but back then I was simply grateful for the attention.

My split with Stuart coincided with another change in my circumstances. I grew bored of life stuck out in the sticks and, with only one bus service a week into Elgin, I felt cut off from civilisation.

Once I gave up my job and lodgings, my options for a home were limited. Out of work, out of pocket and without a roof over my head, there was only one place I could turn – back to Dufftown. Although Rob had still kept on the house, he was no longer there. He had moved to Huddersfield, in West Yorkshire, to be with his new love, Jean, a divorcee. The couple had met during one of her frequent trips to the town to visit her sick father. Responsible also for her mother in England, Jean's loyalty was split and she tried as best she could to divide her time north and south of the border.

Dad and her had clicked instantly and, shortly after they became an item, Rob introduced her to me at a specially arranged lunch in Elgin. I found her pleasant and friendly but, more importantly, it was great for dad to be with someone after the hurt he had suffered with mum's departure.

Although he had decided to move to Huddersfield, where Jean was spending most of her time, he elected to keep on Scorrybreck. It had been our family home for so many years and, because their future plans were unclear, it seemed unnecessary to sell up at that time.

When it became clear I was short of a place to stay, dad immediately offered me the house. Jean and he would return once a month but otherwise the house was empty. I would have the run of the five-bedroom house. I did not take long to make a decision!

Averil, by that time, was studying nursing at The Robert Gordon University in Aberdeen. Living in the city during term-time, she returned to Scorrybreck in the holidays.

Although we hadn't lived under the same roof for nearly two years, we soon resumed hostilities after the enforced ceasefire. As usual, you could not put your finger on a particular reason for our constant bickering, it just happened – in the same way cats will chase mice, so my younger sister and I would nip and moan, and scratch and whine with each other, ad infinitum.

With mum and dad now living in separate countries, it was obvious their days as a couple were over, but the full-time whistle finally blew on their eighteen-year marriage in October that year, when the local sheriff granted the divorce.

Two months from then, I would be twenty-one. As the day approached, dad offered to throw a party for me, mindful that, way back in hospital twelve years previously, it was a landmark none of the medics really believed I would see. As the big day approached, I remained convinced that celebrating was the last thing I wanted to do. What did I have to be cheerful about? My mother lived in a foreign country, my dad lived in England with his new partner, I was once again single, with little prospects of finding a man and I was out of work.

Yes, twenty-one years into my life, and I could not really say that everything was going according to plan.

Dad and Dorothy would have none of it. A party there would be and, miserable or not, I would be there.

Chapter Twenty-six
Twenty-one Candles

Typical, I thought. My birthday, this year, would be Friday the 13th – a cursed day for a cursed life. Magic.

The Commercial Hotel, a fine old hostelry in the town centre, would be the location for my party.

It was fair to say, before that day, I was a "glass-half-empty" kind of girl, someone who would strain to look past the silver linings because I would be convinced a rain cloud was just over the horizon. Now that you've read a fair amount about my life, you might think I had good cause to be pessimistic. I might have an extended family that would put the Royal family to shame but, as far as I knew, Lady Luck was not one of them.

As the invitation replies came back I paid more attention to the no-shows rather than who would actually be there. There would be no Cilla Black-style surprise appearance from mum, no sign of my relatives on Skye.

I went through the motions of trying to be happy about the party. On the day before I visited the local tanning salon for a nice bronzed look and treated myself to a set of fake nails. I looked the part of someone about to enter adulthood, but inside I was in torment.

However, despite my dark mood, something happened that night to wake me from my moroseness. I wouldn't exactly call it an epiphany but, as the party sparked into life, I looked around the assembled throng and realised that I *was* the lucky one.

The people who were not there, for whatever reason, didn't matter to me. Most likely they had all been there for me at some point when I had needed them most. And the family and friends who did attend were among the most important people in my life, my closest allies. Even my long-suffering GP, Dr Heneghan, made it; someone I owed as much to as the surgeons who held my fate in their hands.

As I blew the candles out on my birthday cake that night, the heat from the flickering flames warmed my face. God, I thought, there is a lot here – each one of them seeming to symbolise the second chances I'd been given. As the last candle was extinguished, I made my wish. Convention dictates I cannot say what it was here or, as everyone knows, it will not come true but it was full of hope.

Suddenly it hit me that but for the expertise of my doctors, by rights, I should not have lived beyond the age of four. In another life, I could have been Casey Holter, whose life was cut short by hydrocephalus. I could have been Caroline Nicol. I could have been one of the many other children whose lives were extinguished long before they were allowed to leave anything more than a faint footprint on history.

As the tears welled up in my eyes, I also looked at the twenty-one candles, now no longer flickering flames of gold, and thought of all the youngsters I shared Ward Four with in Aberdeen's Sick Children's Hospital; but especially the ones whose funerals mum attended.

None of them were blessed enough to feel the heat from twenty-one candles on their face, none of them were able to look round a sea of smiling faces and realise they were all here for them.

That night I vowed to change, to never again feel sorry for my lot in life. Sure, I might not have a man to share my life with but that did not mean I had to be lonely. Surrounded by people who loved me, how could I possibly feel down? From that moment, I made a promise to myself to live life to the full; to seize the day and, like mum before me, to recognise happiness when it looked me in the face and act upon it.

After the cake cutting, I made a speech. Despite being some-one who could talk for Scotland, when it comes to having something to say, I clam up. I grabbed the microphone and tried my best to put into words the thoughts racing through my mind. In the end, from what I remember, all that came out was "thanks".

Thanks for being there for me, thanks for pulling me through the trauma I'd suffered since I was a little girl. Just thanks. It didn't matter that I didn't go further than that. Inside my head, I knew what I meant and knew what I had to do.

159

The 13th December 2002 would be a red-letter day in the life of Caroline Macdonald.

That night was also a significant one in the life of a Paisley boy called David Sneddon. The young singer-songwriter triumphed in the BBC's first reality TV talent school show called Fame Academy. His progress through the rounds had me transfixed. Seeing him singing for his survival each week resonated with me. I recall one night, while we were held up in Aberdeen Royal Infirmary for a routine scan. The television was on in the communal waiting area. Hearing him perform a version of the classic Elton John hit "Don't Let the Sun Go Down on Me" moved me. His determination inspired me.

Following his success on the night of my birthday – and in keeping with my newfound resolution to act on impulse – I made it a mission to meet him. The fact he was an absolute heart-throb had nothing to do with it, of course!

Digging out my old contact number for the reporter at the Scottish Sun, which had taken on my negligence case against Moray Docs, I told her about the impact David had on my life.

The bottom line of the story – singing sensation helps tumour girl – clearly ticked the relevant boxes with the top-selling tabloid, which immediately endeavoured to help.

Thinking the best I could get out of the situation was a signed photo, I was stunned when, while sitting at home in Scorrybreck on Hogmanay, just three weeks later, the phone rang. It was David! At first I did not believe it was him and reckoned it was Harry winding me up. Then, to my astonishment, David started singing down the phone to me – the same Elton John number he'd performed so well during the heats of the show. He took my breath away. I couldn't believe someone like him, the nation's man of the moment, had taken time out to speak to me. With incredible charm, he asked about my condition and what it meant for me. It was years since a stranger had taken such an interest in me. By the time he invited me down to meet him at his homecoming concert the following month, you could have knocked me over with a feather. True to his word, David arranged for me to join him in Paisley. I felt like a VIP when, after his show, he approached us, giving me a huge bear hug.

160

For something like this to happen so soon after I'd pledged to make the most of my life was amazing. The special privileges did not end there, however. When David, who went on to secure a number one hit with his self-penned debut single, joined his fellow Fame Academy finalists for a UK tour, Averil and I were invited to Aberdeen for the gig. Once again, we were the ones treated like stars, meeting the entire cast. Blessed with incredible natural talent, their stories inspired me. Often my own clumsiness made me wonder if I had a skill for anything other than survival, yet, possibly, that was something they could relate to.

Like Robert Young, of Cancer Research, before him, David's kindness touched me. Speaking as someone suffering from an incurable condition, I cannot overestimate the benefit children in that situation get from moments like these. The chance to be taken out of your often gloomy, day-to-day existence for a glimpse of celebrity life is all it takes to lift your mood for days, even weeks after. Since meeting him, I've followed David's career with keen interest, always saving a special place in my heart for him.

A further piece of good news followed swiftly after. Mum announced she was coming home for good. Her two-year stint in Spain had been a hard toil but a successful one. Gordon and she had turned around the fortunes of two caravan parks but both felt the time was right for a return to their homeland.

Since they had been away, Robina and Dorothy had given birth to two grandchildren each, and there were more to celebrate on Gordon's side. The thought of missing the key milestones in the youngsters' lives was too much for mum to bear. Hiring a van, they loaded up with all their belongings and headed up the long road back from southern Spain to northern Scotland.

The fact they were coming back to Morayshire delighted me. Although I had managed to visit them twice while they were away, I missed mum terribly. Knowing mum was only a few miles up the road made me feel safe. No one understood me better than she did.

Moreover, when they moved to a new house in Lossiemouth, I had a ready-made place to crash for the night if I was out with friends!

Chapter Twenty-seven
Hello, I'm Sonia

The positive reaction from my meetings with David Sneddon lived with me for weeks. Energised with good feeling, I decided the next step in shaking me out of my doldrums was to get out there and once again test the dating market.

I probably should have learned my lesson with Stuart but, I headed for Downtown, the pub where we'd met, in the hope it might prove a happy hunting ground. Knowing full well I would sit until closing time waiting for someone to buy me a drink, I once again scoured the bar for someone to target.

I must have a sixth sense that enables me to spot an RAF man from fifty paces. My opening gambit this time was as inspired as it was with Stuart. On this occasion, I complemented a stranger on his choice of jeans, adding that they were the same as mine. Not put off by the suggestion he shopped in Dorothy Perkins, the man, Neil, responded favourably. Then, to my astonishment, he offered to swap numbers at the end of the night. Thinking this particular bar must give me special pulling powers, I was oblivious to the reality that it was more likely a regular meat market for desperate servicemen.

Three years older than me and based at Lossiemouth, Neil once again gave me all the early signals that he was a prince among men.

We settled quickly into a routine, which at the time I thought nothing of but to everyone else it immediately raised eyebrows. Every weekend was the same – we'd meet at a popular chain pub for lunch. He would buy the drinks, leaving me, the jobless one, to pick up the tab for the food. Then we'd go off to the cinema. Occasionally he would spend the night but, in-between, I hardly saw or heard from him.

He liked to keep me at arm's length. Unlike Stuart, he refused to tell me where on the base he lived. I dared not take him back to mum's at night so, the only option for him to stay over was in Dufftown.

Incredibly, he would turn up, not only with his overnight bag, but with his empty lunchbox, which he expected me to fill with food I'd paid for.

This went on for two months. Then one evening he plucked up the courage to say what had been on both our minds since day one. It wasn't working out, he said. We were incompatible. If someone had said those words to me at any point during the previous few years, I would have crumpled into a heap and my self-esteem would have hit rock bottom. Not so now. I was simply grateful him saying it spared me the need to make the first move.

As he drove me back to Dufftown that night, I was already planning my next move, thinking where I could go next weekend to help me get back in the saddle, so to speak. Then, as we pulled in to the driveway, Neil turned to me and said: "Let me stay tonight. You know, you're cute in your own funny way. Let's give it another shot."

"Great," I thought. "That'll mean I'm going to have to foot the bill for more lunches."

Sure enough, for another month, we carried on, the same routine as before. Finally, he had enough conviction to put our relationship out of its misery. Relieved it was over, I immediately started to put it behind me but not before indulging in a little retrospective analysis.

Call it women's intuition, but I was convinced he had cheated on me. Just like Stuart, never at any point did I feel like Neil's girlfriend. He seemed happy to use me for whatever pleasure I gave him. My suspicions were confirmed two years after we split up when I bumped into his new girlfriend. Out of curiosity, I asked how long she and Neil had been together. I know I'm not the world's greatest maths genius, but when she said three years, you didn't have to be Einstein to know that our dates overlapped.

Again, a discovery like that would have sent me into therapy not that long ago. Now, I could see our time together for what it was. Although our relationship was never likely to threaten the UK's reigning "Mr and Mrs" champs, Neil provided me with basic security and, for a while I appreciated that. To show how low my self-esteem was before we met, the simple fact I had a man who answered my phone calls was enough to send me to sleep at night contented. However, at the time we parted, I knew I deserved more from a partner. I just hoped I wouldn't have to wait long to find one who cared for me.

A month after meeting Neil, I decided to take steps to put another piece of my life in order. Desperately in need of financial independence, I set about finding work. With the list of unsuitable occupations growing by the year, I wanted something different. Flicking through the pages of a women's magazine, an advert caught my eye. Offering flexible hours, the opportunity to work from home and the benefit of working when I chose, it seemed like my dream job. The only clue to the job description was the term "telephone operator". Intrigued, I rang the number. The reality of the job at first took me by surprise but then fascinated me. It was a sex chatline.

"What the hell," I thought and, with a certain appreciation of the task ahead, wondered, "How hard could it be?"

The parameters were straightforward. When I wanted to work, I just rang up and entered a pin number to alert the switchboard I was online. Then, they would re-route the calls to my home phone number. All I had to do was sit back and wait for the phone to ring. The first thing that surprised me was the volume of calls. I had not appreciated how many perverts were out there.

My bosses gave me a manual to work from but quickly I found it was more fun making up personalities on the spot.

My favourite alter ego was Sonia. I loved her. She was everything I wasn't. Stunning, with flowing natural blonde locks, she was a size eight, when, in reality I was a fourteen. While I was stuck with one blue eye and one green, Sonia had two piercing aquamarine peepers. Mostly she was a highly-sexed nurse, who struggled to keep her clothes on for any length of time but sometimes she'd switch jobs between calls – a policewoman one night, a frisky Wren the next. Older and more worldly-wise than me, Sonia was adept at twisting men round her little finger. Where I was a walking doormat for men to trample over, my other personality was a vixen who kept men dangling, begging for more.

There were no ground rules. I could go as far as I wanted with a caller or cut him stone dead if he became too creepy. They warned me about the nutters I could expect and gave advice on how to deal with child pranksters or men with sick attitudes. Mainly, though, the advice was the same. Regardless of how disgusting the customers were, I needed to keep them on the line for as long as possible. The pay was fine and I could work anytime I wanted. Some weeks I would work two to three hours a night. Evenings were always the busiest time. One minute I'd be watching Coronation Street, the next I'd be purring down the line like a Scottish Eartha Kitt. The majority of callers were pathetic losers on for a quick thrill.

Occasionally though, I would take a call from a lonely old man for whom talking dirty was the last thing on his mind. I felt sorry for these people. I could not imagine being so lonely, my only source of comfort was speaking to a woman I was paying to talk to me. Often they just wanted to chat about themselves, maybe talk about a wife who had died, or workmates who did not understand them. In those circumstances, I just let them talk away, peppering the conversation every so often with some carefully placed "Uh-huhs" and "Is that rights?"

What surprised me was how most men wanted me to describe in great detail what I was wearing, then demanded I take it off as quickly as possible.

The cash allowed me to buy some new clothes and, perhaps, pay for a lunch or two with Neil.

However, I quickly grew tired of having the same dirty chat every night and began looking for a career change.

Another factor hastened my decision to pack in the sex line and kiss goodbye to Sonia. After dumping Neil, I needed a real man to talk to, not the weirdos at the end of the phone.

In June 2003, Cupid finally smiled on me and presented me with the real man I was looking for.

Chapter Twenty-eight
Love is in the Air

He was standing staring in a shop window when I first saw him. Looking resplendent in his blue air force uniform, complete with hat, he stood out instantly from the other Saturday Elgin shoppers.

Like a dream, the thoughts I'd had as I blew out the candles on my twenty-first birthday cake came flooding back.

"Don't let a chance of happiness pass you by Caroline," my inner voice seemed to say.

Almost immediately my old pessimistic self drowned out any words of hope.

"What about those previous losers? How do you know this bloke, even if he does give you the time of day, will treat you differently?"

It was a fair argument. How could I know? Still, nothing ventured, nothing gained. Without even a stiff drink for Dutch courage, I bit the bullet and approached him.

"Didn't I see you out last night?" I offered.

The RAF man looked down at me.

"You what?"

"I saw you out last night," I said, knowing full well I had spent Friday night in the house watching trashy television. "We were in the same pub. We were chatting at the bar."

Luckily for me, he had been out the previous night and came home so worse for wear he could have been discussing the merits of Christmas with Santa Claus and would have been none the wiser.

"Oh aye?" he countered, "Right enough."

I introduced myself. He was Richard, an RAF aircraft technician, seven years older than I was – continuing my trend for older men.

Luckily, my impulsiveness had caught him off guard. That would only get me so far. If I managed to sustain the momentum my opening approach had earned me, we might have something here.

I need not have worried. Conversation came naturally. He was charming, without being smug, confident but not arrogant. We were getting on so well, I was even unsure about playing my T-card. Normally, I get the tumour out there as quickly as possible. I thought the ability to handle information like that separated the men from the boys. This time though, something urged me to hold back. There was no need for shock tactics.

After a healthy chat, we exchanged numbers and made tentative plans to meet. To my delight, I did not have long to wait. The following day Richard rang. He wanted to take me out on Sunday, offering to pick me up from mum's house in Lossiemouth. He came across as even more of a gentleman than his first impression had hinted.

Things were going too well obviously – time for my big mouth to strike again. As Richard pulled up at the house, there were a million and one things I could have said. So why then, for some inexplicable reason, did I come out with, "You've not ironed your shirt."

The look on Richard's face said it all. It was clear he had taken a great deal of time over his appearance. My follow up wasn't much better.

"You look older without your uniform on."

For a split second, I thought he would turn on his heel, get back into his car and drive off. The fact that he didn't probably still causes him consternation to this day.

I'm only grateful he's easy-going because he gave me a second chance. We eventually left the house and, like the day before, spent the night engaged in conversation. The chat flowed between us, instead of the awkward silences that can pollute early dates.

Only when I was sure he was genuinely interested in me did I then mention my health history. Normally the revelation that I live on a knife-edge and could potentially drop dead at any moment gets a reaction, usually along the lines of reaching for a coat and heading for the nearest exit. Richard took it all in his stride. Intrigued by the girl in front of him, his only concern was whether he should have a team of medics on constant call or a speed dial to a brain surgeon on his mobile.

I found it refreshing to talk to someone who listened. Often, when out with older men, I performed the role of listener, my ears bent by tales of their service. This was different. The only fear I had, as we were so comfortable in each other's company, was that we would bypass the lover stage and downshift to being simply friends.

While the bond we were developing was great, I couldn't help thinking, "Is he ever going to kiss me?"

When I thought about previous first dates I'd had, I realised one of the advantages of awkward silences was that you invariably just started snogging to blot out the pauses. So far, during the evening, there had been little opportunity for physical affection.

Referring to my recently rewritten mental guide to life, I realised this was yet another time I would have to deal with the problem directly, lest the opportunity pass me by.

Eventually, I interrupted him.

"Excuse me, could you put your drink down a minute please?" As he placed his glass on the table, I reached over and we kissed for the first time.

The night went so well we agreed to meet up the following day. Over the following week we met up again and again. Throwing caution to the wind, after six days, I asked him to move in with me. Reckless and impulsive, yes, but instinctively it felt right. Practically, it wasn't such a harebrained scheme. Living in that big house all on my own in Dufftown, I welcomed the company. Plus, we were spending so much time in each other's company, it seemed ridiculous for him to drive the thirty miles back to Lossiemouth every night, or morning.

I asked Rob, who was happy, so long as my new lodger contributed to the electricity meter.

Richard thought of it as an adventure. Making the choice between sharing with five RAF men, eating in a communal mess, or living in the relative luxury of a five-bedroom home was surprisingly easy.

The contrast with Neil couldn't have been greater. Richard was happy to put his hand in his pocket where the food was concerned and did not expect me to make his sandwiches. I did it anyway, but out of pleasure not necessity.

169

The more I told him about my condition, the more I felt I could rely on him in a crisis. He seemed genuinely concerned about my epilepsy and, on the rare occasion I fell victim to a panic attack or seizure, he was there to help me out of it.

He was shocked when he first saw me have a seizure but I think he was prepared for something more traumatic than it was. I was at home watching TV, when I blanked out for a few moments. I could hear him talking to me but was frozen, unable to respond. Rather than get freaked out by it though, he was happy he had experienced it. After that, he knew what was required.

These days, he can sense when I am about to have one and prepares for them. It gives me a lot of confidence when we're out together, especially in nightclubs where the flashing lights can sometimes set me off.

After four months it seemed the natural step was to commit to each other. I'd love to be able to say Richard, being a hopeless romantic, surprised me by taking me to the spot we first met before going down on one knee and proposing. The reality was I badgered him for weeks until he finally relented and let me choose the ring I wanted.

At the time of our engagement, there was nothing I wanted more than to wed my Richard. I thought, given the nature of our relationship, that I would be walking up the aisle in months. However, in the short period after Richard placed a ring on my finger, my opinion of marriage flipped on its head. First, dad tied the knot with Jean in Huddersfield. Although invited, I declined to attend. At the time I was sensitive to negative vibes about mum and did not feel comfortable enough to make the trip down south. Then, within three months of each other, Archie married Anne and mum wed Gordon in Lossiemouth.

In the space of a year, my two dads and mum each married for the third time.

Suddenly I did not need a piece of paper to tell me I was in love. Don't get me wrong, I was delighted my parents had found happiness but they would be the last people the government would hire to promote the institution of marriage.

Instead, we decided to move in to our own place and, in April 2004, ten months after we met, we rented a flat in Lossiemouth.

Attempting to contribute to the household income, I landed a job at a local gift shop at weekends. Although I stuck at it for ten months, it was interminably dull. Sometimes I had to wait four hours for a customer. Eventually we decided it was not cost-effective and, because it ate into the only time I have together with my love, I decided to pack it in.

Nowadays, I am practically a housewife, save for the few hours a week when I clean at a local theatre. The situation works for us. For the first time in my life I can say I am truly happy.

Although Richard and I are, in many ways, poles apart, we do compliment each other. I need my home comforts and, on the days when my condition still leaves me shattered, like to stay close to base so I can take a nap when needed. Richard, on the other hand, is always on the go. He loves his high-performance racing bikes, relishes his outdoor pursuits and regularly goes skiing, sailing and cycling. Whenever he has tried to involve me in his activities, it usually ends in disaster.

On one occasion recently, we went camping on the sand dunes near our flat, just to give me a taste of the outdoor life. Richard pitched the tent and, the minute it was up, I dived inside. While he then sparked up the stove, cracked open a few beers and set about rustling up some dinner, I sat freezing inside the tarpaulin. By 2am, I had suffered enough. Storming out of the tent, I demanded he drive me home. Richard, complaining he was over the limit, refused point-blank. Daring me to go, he thrust a torch in my hand and said, "There you go, walk home."

I did, defiantly, striding back over the dunes to our warm flat. I'm sure that night, each of us tried to claim a moral victory. However, it's a perfect example of how Richard treats me as an equal. Fully understanding my limitations, he knows how far he can push me when I need motivation but also recognises the times to put a loving arm around me.

My family were delighted when my relationship with Richard took off – probably because he took some of the emotional burden off them! They hold him in high regard. In fact, after everything I've put my loved ones through, they no doubt think he's the one with the brain disorder, for coming anywhere near me.

I hate to place so much faith in the love of just one person but, before I met him, I did not realise the hope and joy having the support of someone gives you.

For too long, I have been the tumour girl.

My previous boyfriends saw the illness, not the girl. Richard sees past that.

It sounds clichéd but he is truly the man of my dreams. Ever since I was a little girl, I longed for someone to protect me, to care for me like he does. With him, I feel I can do anything. He might be powerless to remove the tumour growing inside my brain but his love for me ensures the world outside is a perfect place to be.

I may have had to kiss a few frogs on the way but, at last, I found my prince.

Epilogue

I believe everything happens for a reason. It took me a long time to reach that philosophical place, though.

Since the doctors discovered my brain tumour, I prayed for one thing – to cut it out. I believed removing it would transform me into a normal child. I blamed its presence for everything that was wrong in my life. It was responsible for my failure at school, my loneliness and my parents' divorce. Of course, these things were all episodes that can happen to any child.

I believed I was different. In reality, I was just the same. I wanted to be normal but I have no idea what normal is. I reacted terribly. I wish I could say I used my setback to become a better person but that's not the case. I focused on the worst-case scenario and, even more terrible, I used the tumour to get what I wanted.

I'm not proud of the way I behaved but I believe I had to go through that process to get where I am today. Where I am is a place where, at last, I've accepted my fate. Now, I believe the tumour defines me. If a medical breakthrough produced a way to remove it, I would miss it.

Accepting it was the turning point in my life. Once I learned to deal with my situation, I felt I could tackle anything. I might not be a doctor, or someone who saves lives on a daily basis, but I found happiness and, in this life, what is more important than that? For too long I spent my time wondering when my life would end, rather than planning when it would start. Yet, as I have grown older, I have come to accept the part my tumour has played in my life and, in the same way that it depends on me to survive, now I believe, in some small, strange way, that I need its continued presence to exist. We have become odd and, for many years, reluctant bedfellows but we get on and, as long as neither of us gets too aggressive with the other, perhaps we can live in harmony for many years to come.

I'm convinced my death sentence could actually become my life sentence.

Many people may raise eyebrows at this somewhat screwball analysis of my situation. However, I have also realised that, while my tumour may yet have a fatal part to play in my future, I am one of the lucky ones. This condition is a lottery. No one determines who lives and who dies. The best you can do is to place your faith in doctors and hope for a way out.

And you have to thank your lucky stars for the most important things. Today, I'm still with my Richard, whose love and support helps put everything in perspective. For years, I never believed I could find a husband to love me, and any thoughts of family were for other people to dream about, not me. Yet now, my surgeon says that with close monitoring, having children is not beyond me. I can live a normal life after all. I still have a lot of growing up to do before I think about any of that but for the first time I am daring to dream of a happy future; and that's good enough for me.